HOW I HEALED MY ULCERATIVE COLITIS: The Cause of Your Illness Is Also the Cure

by NICOLE CARTER, MEd CHES

HOW I HEALED MY ULCERATIVE COLITIS: The Cause of Your Illness Is Also the Cure

NICOLE CARTER, MEd CHES

First Edition

Printed in the United States of America

First Printing, 2022

ISBN 978-0-578-36273-1

For my mother,
who taught me the importance of natural health
at a young age and lit the fire for wellness
that has been with me my whole life

QUIZ: IS THIS BOOK RIGHT FOR YOU?

Do you experience the discomfort of a bloated stomach almost every day? YES / NO

Do you have trouble falling asleep or staying asleep? YES / NO

Do you often feel anxious or experience depression? YES / NO

Do you have low energy throughout the day? YES / NO

Do you have skin irritation, acne or rashes? YES / NO

Do you have joint pain or unexplained body pain? YES / NO

Do you have low nutrient levels such as Vitamin D? YES / NO

Do you have trouble with low testosterone? YES / NO

Do you have irregular periods? YES / NO

Do you have trouble maintaining a healthy weight? YES / NO

If you answered "Yes" to more than 3 of the above you need this book

PART I | MY STORY

ONE: THE SICKEST "HEALTHY" PERSON

For most of my adult life, I have been consumed by a quest for health. I don't know what drives me, but for the past 30 years, I have had a deep interest or preoccupation with health. I have always been in search of learning the best ways of being healthy and have pursued it in my work life as well. I have come to the conclusion that health is simply the *absence of disease*.

It took me a long time to learn that the things that compromise our health not only come from the outside, but also from within. Many factors contribute to sickness, but ultimately most of them have an effect on our gut health which in turn impacts our overall health. Yes, lifestyle choices like diet and exercise have huge impacts, but so does our mental health. Stress, trauma, and what our physical bodies encounter every day will make or break our health.

I'm going to share with you my story of health, disease, and learning. This is my story, but I think it relates to the lives of many. Maybe even yours...

My Health Growing Up

I believe I have lived a very healthy life. I grew up in a small town in Michigan. Like many parts of the Midwest,

Michigan has earned its reputation for natural beauty, and I have very fond memories of growing up in the country and spending most of my time on farmland or on one of the beautiful lakes every summer.

We lived in the city, but my grandparents had an eighty acre farm nearby. My parents divorced when I was five, so my mom would often go back to the farm where she grew up and take us with her. We would spend most weekends visiting the farm, helping my grandparents. I loved going there. Farms were playgrounds for kids before the Internet came along. We would shoot trout in the stream, play hide and seek in the tall cornrows, swing on the ropes in the barns over the cows, and pick herbs and flowers in my grandmother's garden.

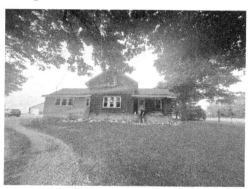

I sometimes rode on my grandfather's combine tractor, watching it clear the rows of plants. We fed the cows on huge grain troughs, and the calves would be fed formula in a bottle - my favorite chore. Farms are rough and dangerous places, and most people today, myself included, would be nervous around all the big animals and heavy machinery. It gave me a certain kind of grit, though, and tremendous respect for nature and raising food.

The farm was such a beautiful place. For many years it was where we learned where food came from. It was not uncommon to drink warm milk freshly milked from the cow, a layer of cream forming at the top as we drank. We often ate homemade baked bread, jam, meat, and milk while at the farm.

Life on a farm is pretty simple for kids, at least it used to be. For me, it was the iconic two-story farmhouse with cracks in the walls on a huge plot of land. A few farm animals, cats and dogs, and a small kitchen garden made up the farm. This was midwestern farmland in the most basic sense. A farmer and his family do all the work with the help of a couple of tractors. It's hard work with little pay but the beauty of farmland is irreplaceable.

Summers were spent making and eating jam. My grandfather would disappear into the fields or barn for hours - or even an entire day. My grandmother would come in to cook the meals or make tea. The long Michigan days seemed to go by so slow in a sleepy farm town. Nothing too exciting except the harvest of the spearmint fields on the neighbor's land that would flood the air with the scent of Wrigley's gum.

In the winter, there was less to do but we still visited the animals in the barn, built snowmen, and baked bread. Looking back, it seems surreal, something from hundreds of years ago instead of just forty.

At the end of each day, we always made our way back to the little town where we lived, thirty minutes from the farm. As we got older, we spent less and less time at the farm. It began to be sold off in parcels as a subsidized farm when my grandparents became too old to maintain the large animals. Eventually, it became a soybean and corn farm with just a few cats running around. By the time I was thirteen, we almost never visited the farm any longer, and my mom had a falling out with her family after my grandmother passed away. When I was fifteen, my grandfather passed away, and the farm was sold to developers. I never set foot on the farm again.

We lived in a little duplex, in the cutest little town called Grand Ledge. I actually loved growing up in this little town, but the lifestyle wasn't the same as on the farm. The food was different, and we didn't spend as much time outside as we did on the farm (though nothing like now). It was quiet and safe, and there wasn't much trouble to find with my mom working all of the time. It was a low-stress, simple life. My mom worked so we walked to and from school each day, returning home to an empty house and looking out for ourselves until Mom got home from work.

Back then, kids like us were called "latch key" kids, and it was the only thing I knew. My mom had to support three kids on a very low salary, so there was no one home to do the after-school homework and prepare the meals for school-aged kids. We managed though, and I became a great cook in the process. I learned to cook all sorts of foods on the stove for myself when I was in grade school. Nothing I made was particularly healthy, but fairly easy to make such as Mrs. Grass Noodle Soup on cold winter days, instant mashed potatoes and of course, pasta. We also loved popcorn, and ate it almost every day if not after school, then as an evening snack. Foods that were inexpensive and easy to make were a good fit for low income families like mine.

I always recognized the difference between the food at my grandparents' farm versus what we ate in the city. The milk was the pasteurized version from the store. The bread wasn't freshly baked. Farm food was only on the farm. City food came from the grocery store. My mom gave us pasteurized skim milk, the "healthier choice", along with the canola oil she used to bake any treats with as opposed to the butter and lard my grandmother cooked with at the farm.

Today, I now know canola oil is simply a waste product that is toxic to humans, and the saturated fat in milk is the best kind of fat to consume. It was during this time, in the '80s, that low-fat foods were hailed as healthy, and replacing saturated fats with seed oils were considered smart choices.

We spent some weekends with my dad, who was on a whole other level with regards to food and health. Common meals at his house included sandwiches, chips, soda, ice cream, and fast food. He also had HBO and Cinemax with all the R-rated movies my sister and I weren't allowed to watch at my mom's. Weekends at Dad's were full of indulgences. My constant belly aches never seem to be connected to the food, though. Food was just something to eat that should taste good, there was little to no regard for its impact on health or nutritional offering.

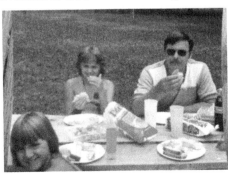

In that time frame, obesity was on the rise, and my dad was certainly contributing. He was a police officer for many years and ate in the way police were often known to do. Donuts and coffee were a daily meal, followed by fast food while on the job and maybe some more fast food on the way home for dinner. My dad was not a big cook, so Taco Bell and Burger King made regular appearances.

My mom and dad were polar opposites when it came to food and nutrition. Mom was very concerned and chose foods for us with the intention of nourishing our bodies. My dad never made that connection for himself or his kids. He was fairly sedentary, smoked and ate a lot of processed and fried foods. Even though he had terrible habits, I believe it was the ongoing everyday stress that he lived with that ultimately caused most of his health problems. He suffered child abuse at the hands of his mother as a young child, served as a Marine in Vietnam and became the most intense workaholic I have ever known. He literally destroyed his own life with his habits, but never seemed to be able to make the behavior changes needed to reset his course. He died at the age of sixty-six from his fourth heart attack.

Stress, Trauma and Health

In 2019 the Centers For Disease Control published the ACE's study, which showed that Adverse Childhood Events significantly impacted one's health as an adult.

The report revealed that about 60% of Americans experienced at least one adverse experience during childhood. Adverse events include physical, emotional, or sexual abuse, physical or emotional neglect, or dysfunctions in the household such as mental illness, violent parent, divorce, family incarceration, or substance abuse.

What they found was that more than 15% of those surveyed had four or more different ACEs. Those with ACEs had an increased risk of chronic disease, obesity, autoimmune disease, and other health risks due to prolonged or excessive stress response. It turns out that the prevalence of ACEs is exceptionally high. Nearly 61% of those surveyed had at least one adverse childhood event, and 1 in 6 had four or more.[1]

I never felt particularly stressed as a kid, but looking back at my life, it was stressful, and I am surprised I didn't have more health problems. I had 6 ACEs as a child, and sadly most of them are pretty standard amongst kids' lives today.

When I was about six years old, my parents divorced, adverse event #1. I have some unpleasant memories about this, but one thing stands out clearly: the numerous illnesses I had after the divorce. I had endured abandonment by my father, had a mother who was forced to work so hard she was never there and was often left to my own devices. My parents fought viciously, and we had to be in court to talk about our lives. For a young kid, this was frightening.

My mom was much calmer than my hothead dad, and even though I loved them both, things were much more peaceful with my mother. She received full custody of us, which also meant my dad was supposed to pay her child support. I don't think he ever did. Mom had a low-paying job and struggled to make ends meet, adding to the stress in our household. Keeping the power on and the refrigerator filled was a challenge. I was well aware of this after having the phone or power turned off on us. Even as a youngster, I had the realization that the electricity could shut off at any time, and this was a scary thing for a kid living in the cold state of Michigan.

We moved out of our family home and into a small townhouse in the city of Grand Ledge, where I would spend the rest of my youth. I loved that town. It was safe and quiet and a great place to raise kids.

However, my childhood was filled with a lot of uncertainty and lacked stability after my parents' divorce. My mom made it work the best she could, but I had far more worries and concerns than any young child ever should.

I didn't realize it at the time, but my years from 5-12 included several adverse events, and my body was responding. At just six years old, I encountered my first trauma of sexual abuse, of which I can recall only parts. Around that time and for years to come, my stomach was always causing me trouble, and I sometimes ended up in the hospital with complaints that doctors could never explain or resolve. I was chronically constipated, bloated, nauseated and uncomfortable, but it just became part of life, and at some point, I stopped complaining to my mom about it. She was not aware of the sexual abuse. It turns out, that sexual abuse in childhood has a significant correlation with irritable bowel syndrome. In one interesting study, sexual abuse appears to be the post-potent contributor to IBS, but emotional and physical abuses can also contribute to the disease, though less distinctly.[2]

You may wonder, why am I sharing all of this very private information with you. The reason is, I know how common stress is, and particularly childhood trauma and abuse. A 2009 meta-analysis of 65 articles covering 22 countries indicated that 19.7% of women experienced sexual abuse before the age of 18, and of men, 7.9%.[34]

In addition, the WHO in 2002 estimated that 73 million boys and 150 million girls under the age of 18 years had experienced various forms of sexual violence.[5]

A more recent study in 2014 claims that 1 in 9 girls and 1 in 53 boys experience sexual abuse from an adult. An appalling number, which based on the data could be a driver of digestive diseases in today's adults.[6]

More specific to my disease, ulcerative colitis, I found some interesting research as well. One population-based study concluded that childhood physical and sexual abuse are related to ulcerative colitis, (but not Crohn's disease) and stated that those who are physically or sexually abused during childhood had significantly higher odds of ulcerative colitis than their non-maltreated peers.[7]

One possible reason this occurs is that when there is trauma to the body or psyche, the vagus nerve may be damaged. The vagus nerve is the tenth cranial nerve that carries an extensive range of signals from the digestive system and organs to the brain and back again to the organs. It innervates (runs through) the stomach and digestive organs. When the vagus nerve is damaged due to trauma, the nerve may not stimulate the organs in the way it should, and as a result digestion could be impaired. In a paper published in 2018 in *Frontiers in Psychiatry*, the vagus nerve represents the main component of the parasympathetic nervous system, which oversees a vast array of crucial bodily functions, including control of mood, immune response, digestion, and heart rate.[8]

Sexual abuse, and any abuse experienced as a child has life long effects that erode health. I share my experience, because it is not something your doctor will ask you when you are diagnosed or even on an initial visit regarding some kind of digestive issue such as IBS or others. *The fact is, abuse is a major contributor, and it must be recognized and addressed.*

When the stress response is turned on due to stressful events or trauma, the body goes into the fight or flight mode, or the sympathetic state. The body can't properly digest the food you have eaten when you are in a sympathetic state. Digestion is not a priority; running and fighting are. So, our digestive fluids slow down, and overall digestion is impaired. It is a common reason why people under stress often have constipation, bloating or acid reflux.

My mom was considered a "health nut" because of her healthy habits. She didn't eat junk food, never drank alcohol, and walked several miles every day. She favored a trip to the chiropractor over the typical child and family "well visit." Mom also didn't let us have any junk food at all, which irritated us. We would be thrilled with a bag of corn chips showing up on the Fridays she was paid.

Most of our meals included chicken or fish, soups, salads, and fruit. She never bought soda or candy. On weekends we would have the special treat of a trip to the Quality Dairy convenience store for a giant ice cream cone for $.50. We could afford that, and my mom had an obsession with ice cream, the only unhealthy food I ever saw her eat. Still, we thought we were starving and would jump at the chance to gobble up any junk food when given the opportunity.

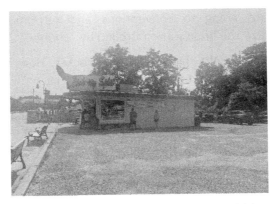

We did not take medications when we were kids, and we had few, if any, vaccinations. My mom would let our bodies work out any bugs with the natural fevers. We used a cold cloth on the head, ginger ale, baking soda baths, and chicken soup for just about every ailment. We were all pretty healthy, rarely were any of us sick, and definitely no chronic illnesses. I often had ear infections, which were resolved when my mom discontinued the dairy. I was given many rounds of antibiotics to resolve those ear infections though at the time there was no consideration for what they might do to one's gut. In fact, the term "microbiome" was not even used until 2001 when it was first coined by microbiologist, Joshua Lederberg.

As we got older, my mother's hunger for health brought her to the path of energy medicine. This was far-fetched "science" in the '80s and no one really took her seriously. Little did they know, Energy Medicine would be defined by the National Institutes of Health in the '90s as an area with Complementary and Alternative medicine. Mom lived and breathed energy medicine. She was constantly reading books and manuals about it. She would spend many weekends going to conventions and retreats, learning about how the body was controlled by "energy."

We all thought she was off her rocker. How could you press on your arm to tell you what is going on within your body? It was absurd. The body can tell you whether something is good or bad for it, she would say. It all seemed like a hoax, but she was convinced, and the rest of our lives were influenced by her passion for health and energy medicine. I later realized that my time pouring over health and nutrition books was not far from my mom's obsession with energy medicine - that she was my initial influence in health.

I followed the typical teenager habits regarding health and nutrition, which is to say I didn't care much. I did start running around age thirteen, however, and was always very active. I ran track in school and was on the dance team as well. In Michigan, it is common for people to be relatively sedentary. Luckily I was active, and that probably helped to offset my less healthy food choices.

When I was sixteen, I spent a summer in Denmark living with a host family. The father in that family was a runner as well. Even though he didn't speak English, he would put the stopwatch on my wrist and point me in the direction to run. I ran many miles that summer and learned how the Danish enjoyed food, family, and beer. When I got home to Michigan, I was a new person. I had seen another part of the world and was ready to DO SOMETHING. I quit the dance team and got a job. I had wanted a car, so I could have as much freedom as I did in Denmark. Running took a back seat, and work and saving money became my only interests.

After graduating high school, I took my first year at the local community college because I received a grant to attend that year for free. I had no idea what I wanted to do, but I was anxious to leave the tiny town that I grew up in and spread my wings. I finished the year and immediately moved to Las Vegas, where my dad lived. I found a roommate and proceeded to spend my first college year there as most college students do. I attended classes during the day, waiting tables in between classes and in the evening. After work, I would party until the early morning hours, only to wake up and repeat it the following day. We would often end our nights with breakfast at one of the all-night greasy spoon Vegas diners. On the weekends, I crammed and tried to catch up on my studies, but my grades were suffering, and I was the unhealthiest I had ever been in my life.

On Halloween, I got dressed up to go to a party and found that the cat costume that I had been planning no longer fit. It suddenly occurred to me that I had gained weight with the lifestyle I was living. I didn't feel good physically, and I didn't feel good about the way I looked. That was enough to flip the switch, and I began to run again.

As the weight started coming off, I found more interest in food and how it affected my health. It was the first time in my life I had made the connection between my body and what I ate. I found a diabetic meal plan that I had intended for my dad and decided to try it myself. It was a low-carb diet, the first I had ever tried. I was astonished when I quickly dropped 20 pounds in what seemed like a matter of weeks. I was so excited and intrigued that I decided to pursue a career in health and nutrition. I became an ACSM certified personal trainer and fell in love with the health and fitness industry. I switched from waiting tables to personally training while finishing college. I eventually graduated with my Bachelor's degree in psychology, but I had already discovered that this was not the direction where I wanted my career to go. I was now going full tilt into the health and wellness industry, which felt like home.

At this time, I was still practicing veganism, and it was not even trendy at the time. It was considered very extreme and weird. I had done exhaustive research on meat-free diets, found some compelling evidence, and went all in. In hindsight, you can find the motivation was to save the planet by doing the "right thing" by not contributing to the animal agriculture industry, and trashing the environment. I followed a vegan diet for many years and even a raw vegan diet for at least one year. My goal with nutrition was to get the most nutrients in the least amount of calories. I would consider myself a "hippie," always concerned with eating to save the planet while preventing any kind of disease of my own. I figured that if I could eat as many vegetables as possible, there is no way I would encounter any sort of illness or weight issue. I thought that I had it all figured out; this was the path to health.

My vegan diet eliminated all animal products. I would not even eat honey! I continued to eat grains, legumes, fruits, and vegetables as was suggested by the health gurus I had read. I was still just a kid, though, so I often ate baked goods, sugary foods, and drank beer - along with the healthier stuff. I was also a runner at this time, working most of my days and nights waiting tables while going to college. I was losing weight with all the activity, so to me, that meant I was doing things right. "Skinny" was synonymous with "healthy", right?

For a while, this worked pretty well. I did have a few minor health conditions like fatigue, bloating, and headaches but was ultimately doing well - considering the workload and late nights in the city. It wasn't until I had gotten married and wanted to have kids that I started to have health problems. At twenty-five, I began to think about having babies but I was also having irregular periods at this time and they came with painful cramps and extreme fatigue. I learned that I had endometriosis and was told I would never have kids. This was the first indication that my health was not what it seemed.

At twenty-eight, I was in graduate school studying for my Public Health degree. I was preparing for a final exam that would kick off my summer vacation. I was planning on acing my exam, then driving to my favorite beach town in California to spend some time relaxing by the water with my husband, but as I was drinking my coffee and reviewing my class notes, a sudden and intensely sharp pain struck me and brought me to my knees. I thought maybe I was having some kind of severe cramping. I went to the kitchen cabinet to find some pain reliever, and the next thing I knew, I was waking up on the kitchen floor surrounded by bottles and pills from my medicine box.

I had passed out from internal bleeding that I was not even aware was happening. The pain became so severe, I tried to call 911 but was confused about what was happening. I thought I must be overreacting, I called them back and told them I was ok, I was probably just having cramps. I didn't want to be a wimp. I called my husband and told him what was going on. He said to call 911 but I lost consciousness again, waking up to the sound of his voice yelling from the phone. He was in California at the time, with no way to help me. I crawled to the door to unlock it for the paramedics before passing out again. He called his mother and sister, who were only ten minutes from my house. They found me unconscious on the living room rug with the phone in my hand, my husband still on the line. They got me into the car and drove me to the hospital.

Once in the ER, my mother-in-law, a former nurse, demanded someone come out and look at me. I was grey and barely coherent. Finally a doctor came to the waiting room and I was taken in right away. I recall them palpating my abdomen, to which I screamed in pain. After giving me pain medication and some tests, I remember someone saying to me, "Did you know you were pregnant?" I had no idea. Within an hour, I had an emergency tubal ligation to stop the bleeding. I had lost a lot of blood, and needed two blood transfusions, lost one fallopian tube, and the fetus, but I was alive. Once out of the hospital, it took me weeks to regain my strength and energy after the stress my body went through. The loss of blood made me very fatigued, and I was depressed at the thought that I may never have a baby and missed the once chance I may have had. My doctor said not to expect anything, natural pregnancy was not likely with just 1 fallopian tube. Three months later I was graced with a miracle, and despite the odds I was pregnant with my first child.

Being the uber health-conscious hippie that I was, I had both kids at home with no medication. I didn't choose that for a badge of honor (you don't get a medal for giving birth), but I did not trust the medical system. I did not want my babies being given unnecessary interventions unless necessary. At the time my kids were born, it was common practice for hospitals to give some medications immediately upon birth.

I was a natural woman, and I wanted a natural birth with no drugs for either me or my babies. Studying natural health had fully convinced me that modern medicine caused more harm than good. I read The Sanctity of Human Blood by Timothy O'Shea along with other texts about natural immunity from birth, and I trusted my body to do that work. I didn't want any part of it involved with my babies, so I hired a midwife and had the most amazing experiences of my life birthing and raising my children naturally. I wanted to avoid all drugs, and medical interventions, just natural medicine and plant-based diets for us all. My belief in the power of plants and natural healing was strong, and I wanted to keep my family as healthy as possible, so I found creative ways to get as much plant matter in my body as possible, as was my goal. I truly believed in what I was doing. I had no idea the kind of damage I was doing.

Having babies took a toll on me like it does to all women. I felt extreme fatigue, depression, was experiencing hair loss, and found myself cold all the time. I would take my daughter out to play and would harness the few seconds it took her to walk up the ladder and slide down the slide to close my eyes and rest my head down. That was a common trend. I was still a runner, and I could manage my morning run and almost daily yoga, but the fatigue would hit me by mid-day, and the rest of the day and evening was such a struggle.

I continued with the vegan diet, convinced this was the best choice both for me and the planet. I was still drained, had thinning and falling hair, recurrent urinary tract infections, and kidney infections. I was often moody and depressed. Being a mom with very young kids is draining and I attributed the exhaustion to just that. I just could not believe my diet could be the problem. Wasn't a vegan diet the healthiest diet on the planet? I made it a point to eat most of my vegetables raw now because that was their most nutritious state, (or so I thought). I had escalated my cultish thinking to the next level, raw veganism. Everything I ate was a raw vegetable or fruit. I sprouted nuts and seeds and ground them into dips, crackers and desserts. I sprouted grains on occasion and dehydrated them to create all sorts of crackers which I topped with more pate made of nuts or seeds. It was not uncommon for me to have a giant blender full of "green smoothie" each day, consisting of bananas, mangos, and spinach. It doesn't get much healthier than that, right?! Unfortunately, there was so much I didn't know and would not acknowledge about that way of eating. My health continued to spiral, and I became more of an overzealous vegan, thinking I just must not be doing a good enough job.

I was clearly suffering from some thyroid challenges but at the time was not aware. All of my symptoms aligned but more importantly, being on a plant-based diet led me to filling my plates with foods that can really harm that important gland. It turns out that iodine is very toxic to the thyroid, (even though it is commonly believed to be beneficial for thyroid) and is even sold in many health food stores as a dietary supplement to support thyroid health. In addition, tofu, soy products, and cruciferous vegetables can damage thyroid and I was eating them in large quantities - raw - every day.

The foods that are often touted as "superfoods" were actually loaded with goitrogens. To top things off, I was a very big green tea drinker. I drank a quart or more of green tea per day. Despite it being hailed for its EGCG content, it can also reduce thyroid function by increasing TSH levels. This is not good.[9]

In 2010, I came down with pancreatitis, which is usually reserved for alcoholics, though I didn't drink at the time. I never go to the doctor, but this time I called my in-laws to watch the babies so I could take myself to the ER to see what was going on. I was notified I would not be leaving for a while due to elevated liver enzymes and a pancreatitis diagnosis, which can be life-threatening.

I had no idea what was going on, or why. I had a constant deep ache in my abdomen that went clear through to my back. The pain was intense. I couldn't eat anything without feeling immediately nauseated. After several tests, I was told I had a poor functioning gallbladder and "sludge" in there to boot. How was this even possible? How can someone who eats only plants and receives colon hydrotherapy have digestive problems? Do vegans even get illnesses? I had my gallbladder removed shortly thereafter.

Looking back, I know how naïve this was, but I could not make sense of it at the time. I was pretty obsessed with my health and could not imagine anything I was doing could be harming me. One of my friends said something at the time that I have never forgotten. "You are the sickest healthy person I know!"

She was right. I was an extremist with my health, yet I was sick all of the time. The sad part is, it was obvious to other people, but it was not even on my radar. When you really want to believe something is true, THAT is the only truth you will see. You can find research and testimonials to support your cause, or any cause, but that does not make it correct.

I went on to have a variety of other health challenges for years. I struggled with energy, my hair was falling out, I felt depressed and anxious often, and I seemed to get sick with the flu and kidney infections repeatedly.

My chiropractor had me do saliva hormone testing as well as some bloodwork to find out what was going on. It turns out that even living in Las Vegas, NV I had extremely low levels of Vitamin D in my blood as well as very low levels of all my hormones. Based on what I was eating, this made sense. I did not eat meat or dairy products, so I was getting no saturated fats in my diet at all. On top of that I was not getting nearly enough protein, and my vitamin B12 levels were very low, despite having already been supplementing them daily.

My doctor urged me to stop the vegan diet and to at least include eggs, but I was hell bent on making my vegan diet work. Despite the challenges with my hormones, my thyroid, my fatigue and my mood, I was so brainwashed into believing that this diet was everything it took me another year to finally add some animal products back into my diet. I did eventually eat the eggs my doctor suggested and I did feel an improvement. I added fish as well, but continued to eat large amounts of raw vegetables every day.

Even though I felt some improvement in my energy level I often felt bloated and constipated. I assumed that since vegetables were the healthiest foods, the more I could eat of them the better. A common misbelief.

TWO: REACHING OUT FOR HELP

People generally have a very distorted perception of health. Around 2011, I had shifted from traveling with a network marketing job to more fitness and coaching. During this time in my life, I was skinny from extreme dieting and intense exercising. I had started teaching barre and yoga classes daily, something I have always loved to do. When I completed my yoga training, there were a lot of nuances to health and nutrition within the group and in the yoga community as a whole. I never thought about it at the time, but excessive dietary restriction and vegan diet and lifestyle is fairly common. This may come partially from the Hindu roots, but it may also come from the fitness world's influence on diet and restrictive eating habits.

During this time I taught seven to ten classes per week and did some additional walking and jogging on top of that. I was also modeling and felt that I needed to stay thin. It was very intentional. I was a health coach because I loved helping people lose weight and feel better. I had figured out how to do it and I knew how much better I felt after getting rid of some unnecessary body fat.

Losing weight is not that hard, but apparently, being healthy is not equivalent to thinness. People assume "thin" also means "healthy", but it does not. I may have been skinny, but on the inside, my stomach bothered me every day. I felt tired most of the time. I was exercising a lot and eating what I thought was a healthy diet, but my digestive symptoms kept getting worse. I was an emotional wreck on the inside, and a picture of health on the outside. Almost everything I ate at this point seemed to bother my stomach. I was obsessed with health, but not healthy myself. I was unhappy with my life and feeling extremely stressed.

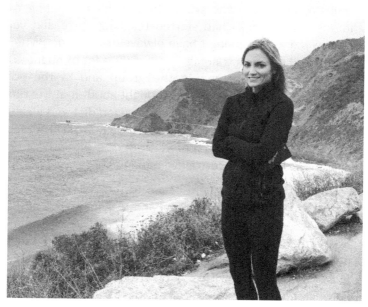

In September of 2012, my dad passed away. He was already in very poor health being obese and diabetic. I knew the end was coming for him, but you can never really be prepared for the death of a parent. My dad was never in good health, in all of my years of memory of him. His lifestyle was conducive to the diseases he was suffering from. He was diabetic, had heart disease and had had 3 prior heart attacks. He ate fast food daily, sat most hours of the day, never exercised, smoked a pack of cigarettes a day, and was a complete workaholic.

Watching him struggle with chronic illnesses fueled my interest in health. His counters were covered with prescription bottles, which he took diligently. Each one seemed to create a new problem for him, though. His issues were nothing a pill could fix. They were deep-rooted issues that required behavior change, not a drug. Unfortunately, he was unwilling to make the necessary changes. He was damaged from trauma, and child abuse and Vietnam had altered his mind making him quite self-destructive, though he never realized that.

His passing was tough for me because it brought back the years of trauma and feelings of abandonment I had lived through as a child myself. My dad's death created intense feelings of regret and sadness that I would never have him in my life, or in my kids' lives. It was a major life stressor for me, as it is for most people with a death in the family.

Soon after my dad's death, my marriage began to crack and crumble. The stress and emotions compounded with the existing struggles and strain on our relationship became too much. My husband and companion of 18 years separated. The division of the family was devastating, and I believe that it contributed to the illness that had long been brewing in me.

I thought I would raise my kids in the idyllic family dynamic. For many years I had what was considered a perfect life. I was very blessed during my marriage and we lived comfortably, had nice things, and took many vacations. Sadly, those things didn't make up for the loneliness I felt. We lived in the desert, which did not offer much of anything that I enjoyed. Looking back, I will admit that I was not living in my truth and was not happy in my marriage, or in my life at all.

My husband was a loving and hardworking man and he had a solid career that provided a lot for us. The career was also what took him away from home much of the time and I often found myself sad and lonely, wishing I had a true partner to enjoy life with. Instead, I was with someone with whom I could not connect due to lack of time and distance. Ultimately, the life I lived was not the one I wanted. My zest for life and optimism for the future was gone, and I felt depressed and depleted. We divorced a year later, and It would be one of the most emotional and stressful times in my life.

After my divorce, I was stuck in depression. I feared the future and didn't want to look at the present. I had no faith in finding a new partner, didn't want to attempt another relationship, and was more worried about how my future with my kids would unfold. I went out most nights when the kids were not with me. Anything to distract me from the emotions I was feeling, but often, they were late nights with a lot of alcohol. I knew I still had to come back to reality in the morning, but I thought if I could keep up the distractions long enough, maybe I could ride out the feelings until it was over.

Although that tactic didn't really work, it did worsen my condition. I could clearly see the symptoms worsen after a night of drinking. I was concerned, but I didn't want to deal with it. It was just one of the many bad things that had happened in my life and I really just wanted to ignore it. My now ex-husband was aware of my condition and urged me to take care of myself, to do something. He would remind me often that if I didn't get a handle on things, I could be putting my life in jeopardy and what would that do to my children? I felt hopeless and powerless, but I wanted to fix it.

I think it is essential to acknowledge that stress is a significant factor in health. I entirely overlooked this at the time. Also, I think it is safe to say that most people do not reach out for help when they feel emotionally stressed - at least not until things get so severe they are forced to deal with a related illness such as depression or cancer. I did not recognize then, nor at any time in my life previous to becoming sick, that stress could have such an impact on my health. It was not taught in much detail in graduate school, where I studied Health Promotion.

Stress management was not talked about much at that time, either. It was not something that the medical field connected to autoimmune disease in any way. It is barely even talked about now by doctors, even though the research is emerging. Yet, we all have stress in our lives, don't we? Some of us even have past traumas that still affect us and our health in the present. I had a childhood filled with trauma, emotional neglect, sexual abuse, abandonment, and loneliness, but I never connected it to my physical health.

Sometimes we don't realize the impact stress has on our health until it becomes visible, and even then, most of us ignore it. That September, it became undeniably visible to me. I had blood in my stool for the first time. Of course, this is very alarming. There are many reasons one can have blood in the stools, but I didn't know any of that. All I knew was that this was not good. I watched closely for a few days, and it never went away. Days soon turned into weeks and I was still bleeding.

Nothing had really changed in terms of how I felt. I had become accustomed to the usual stomachache, fatigue, and bloating. By this point, it was something I had experienced for years. Thinking back, I have had stomach issues since childhood. It was somewhat normal for me to feel this way. I never talked to anyone about it, so in my reality, it was just another day.

Maybe it was fear, or perhaps it was denial, but I had a hard time coming to terms with the fact that something was wrong with me and that I might need some professional help. The fear of what could be going on in my stomach was taking me over, and I needed answers. I wasn't getting any better and had no idea what to do. I didn't know what I was dealing with. I searched the Internet for "blood in stool" and most of it led to: "See your doctor", which I didn't want to do. Often it referred to hemorrhoids, which I had never experienced so I didn't know what to look for. I recall coming across what's referred to as anal fissures, but the descriptions never seemed to apply to me. I was coming up empty-handed.

Before then, I had never heard of ulcerative colitis and was not familiar with Crohn's disease. For once, I couldn't figure out how to deal with a health issue of my own, and that really frustrated me. I was stubborn and wanted to do it my way. All-natural, just like I did with my kids. Whatever it was, I could figure it out. I always worked out my own health issues. After a couple more weeks of stomach pain and bleeding stools, I finally called the doctor to schedule an appointment. I had to admit defeat, and that I couldn't fix this on my own. I didn't even know what I was dealing with. I needed to concede to the medical world in which I had so much distrust. There seemed to be no other options. I decided it was time to address it and to clean it up, even if it required some medication. Either way, it needed to stop.

In October 2012, I reluctantly visited my doctor. He listened to my concerns, gave me an examination to rule out hemorrhoids, and scheduled me for a colonoscopy. What a miserable process it was to prepare for that procedure. I had to fast and drink a horrible liquid I learned was referred to by others as "colon blow," so you can imagine what it does to you. I figured it would all be worth it, though. I would get to the bottom of it, find the cause, and take whatever steps were necessary to fix it. The misery would be temporary, I believed.

A few days after the colonoscopy, I was back in my doctor's office to review the results. I was nervous but so ready to be done with this and was willing to follow instructions even if I didn't agree. He sat next to me with images from the colonoscopy. The pictures showed what looked like the inside of your mouth. It was red tissue, with white spots all over it. It was my colon, covered in hundreds of tiny ulcers. I had no idea what I was looking at, but he showed me pictures of what a healthy colon looked like, and suddenly, I realized mine was very sick. I received a shocking diagnosis that ultimately changed how I would perceive food and health. The healthiest person I knew was now facing a deadly autoimmune disease called ulcerative colitis.

Fear is often the trigger that makes people change their behavior. They may have unhealthy habits, find out from their doctor they are diabetic or have cancer, and suddenly emerge with pristine health habits. I was definitely motivated by fear, but in my case I thought I had nothing to change. I was already living an exemplary healthy life. I ate an enormous amount of vegetables every day, avoided fat, avoided sugar and exercised more than anyone else I knew. How much healthier could I be? There was not much to improve on, I assumed.

I had done everything thus far in my life to prevent being sick and overweight like my dad had been. I thought I had it all figured out, that I knew all there was to know about nutrition and exercise. When it turned out that I was very sick, I was ashamed to admit it to anyone. What did it say about me as a health educator or even a coach? Who wants to take advice from a sick person?

I was not someone to ever ask for help with things and felt like I could handle most anything on my own. After all, I grew up without much support, and I learned it's best not to rely on anyone but yourself. This time, though, it was out of my control. I had exhausted my possibilities and had to ask for help - a very humbling experience. The worst part was that there was not much help (or hope) offered. To me, living off drugs to maintain health isn't "health". It is how medicine has operated for a long time. It isn't healthcare, it's "sick care", and I wanted nothing to do with it.

---

[1]https://www.cdc.gov/violenceprevention/aces/fastfact.html
[2] Sansone, R. A., & Sansone, L. A. (2015). *Irritable Bowel Syndrome: Relationships with Abuse in Childhood. Innovations in*

clinical neuroscience, 12(5-6), 34–37

[3] Noemí Pereda, Georgina Guilera, Maria Forns, Juana Gómez-Benito, *The prevalence of child sexual abuse in community and student samples: A meta-analysis, Clinical Psychology Review*, Volume 29, Issue 4, 2009,Pages 328-338,

[4]https://www.sciencedirect.com/science/article/abs/pii/S0272735809000245

[5] Geneva: World Health organization; [Last cited on 2014 Aug 09]. *Child maltreatment*. Updated 2014.

http://www.who.int/topics/child_abuse/en/ [Google Scholar]

[6] David Finkelhor, Anne Shattuck, Heather A. Turner, & Sherry L. Hamby, *The Lifetime Prevalence of Child Sexual Abuse and Sexual Assault Assessed in Late Adolescence*, 55 Journal of Adolescent Health 329, 329-333 (2014)

[7] Fuller-Thomson E, West KJ, Sulman J, Baird SL. *Childhood Maltreatment Is Associated with Ulcerative Colitis but Not Crohn's Disease: Findings from a Population-based Study. Inflamm Bowel Dis. 2015 Nov*;21(11):2640-8. doi:

10.1097/MIB.0000000000000551. PMID: 26230860

[8] Breit, S., Kupferberg, A., Rogler, G., & Hasler, G. (2018). *Vagus Nerve as Modulator of the Brain-Gut Axis in Psychiatric and Inflammatory Disorders. Frontiers in Psychiatry*, 9, 44.

https://doi.org/10.3389/fpsyt.2018.00044

[9]https://www.ncbi.nlm.nih.gov/pmc/articles/PMC4740614/

THREE: DIAGNOSIS DOOMSDAY

When someone tells you that you have a disease with no known cause or cure, it is reasonable to feel depressed and defeated, there is no hope, and the best you can hope for is "managing" the illness. Since I studied health and nutrition, I was still shocked that this could be happening to me. I was doing everything right. I still believed the cure was in food, and when I asked my doctor what type of diet I should follow, he said, "Diet doesn't matter." What?! How could this possibly be true? Isn't ulcerative colitis a disease of the digestive system?

He proceeded to tell me that as long as I took my medication daily, I had a good chance of keeping my colon for another ten years. Still, unfortunately, many people eventually lose their colon, and some die from colon cancer or infection. Are you kidding me? This disease can't happen to me. I am the healthiest person I know! I took the prescription for pills and suppositories and left the office in tears. I cried all the way home, stunned at what I had just been told. Shock and disbelief were all I could feel. I was angry at my efforts to be healthy all these years, which now proved useless. If that lifestyle was not the answer, what was? I sat with my kids, then 6 and 9, and considered how old they would be in 10 years. Would I be able to work and make a living? I was a single mother; they needed me. How long would I live with this? Would I see them graduate high school? The worst-case scenarios plagued my mind.

Feeling like I had no options, I filled my prescriptions and read up on the possible side effects. One of the prescriptions I was given to control my condition was Lialda or mesalamine. Possible side effects from this drug include rectal bleeding, bloody diarrhea, and stomach pain. Weren't these the exact symptoms I was trying to cure?

The list of other side effects was long. It included bloody urine, blurred vision, chest tightness, dark urine, diarrhea, difficulty breathing, dizziness, fever, bloating, general feeling of discomfort and illness, headache, itching or skin rashes, joint pain, loss of appetite, muscle aches, and pains, nausea, pain around the eyes, pounding in the ears, pressure in the stomach, shivering, slow or fast heartbeat, sore throat, stomach cramps, sweating, swelling of the stomach area, trouble sleeping, tiredness or weakness, vomiting, vomiting of blood and yellow eyes or skin. These were the more common side effects, there were many more listed that could also happen. Was it really possible that this disease could only be treated with drugs that could create a whole host of other symptoms? I couldn't understand how other people just accepted this as the only option.[10]

Ulcerative colitis is often treated with anti-inflammatories, immune system suppressors, and biologics. Most of the anti-inflammatory drugs are either corticosteroids or aminosalicylates either taken orally or as a suppository/enema. Most people get some relief from a flare when using them, however, it really is just a bandaid, and when the drug stops the inflammation usually returns.

Immune system suppressors reduce the inflammatory response but also increase your risk of cancer and heart problems. Biologics such as Humira or Remicade are TNF (Tumor Necrosis Factor) inhibitors that work by neutralizing a protein produced by your immune system. They are usually only used in severe cases when nothing else is working. The last stop, if you will, of the drug world for UC. In addition to these drugs, you may be prescribed antidiarrheals, pain medication, and iron supplements.

I had no idea what to do next or where I would end up. The only thing I could see was years of drugs and side effects until I would end up losing my colon and wearing an ostomy bag for life.

For months, I found myself depressed, going out and drinking at night to avoid thinking about the situation. I felt like the healthy life I lived so far was pointless. I shut down, withdrawing from friends and family. I stopped talking to my sister. I kept two close friends who knew my whole life, and that was it. Everyone else was held at a distance. I knew I was not in a good place. Something had to change.

Common Knowledge About Colitis And Other IBDS, Common Outcomes

Inflammatory bowel disease is an umbrella term used to describe disorders that involve chronic inflammation of your digestive tract but primarily refers to Crohn's and colitis.

Other digestive disorders include irritable bowel syndrome, diverticulitis, gastroesophageal reflux disease, gastroparesis, gastritis, peptic ulcer disease, celiac disease, ulcers, and SIBO (small intestinal bacterial overgrowth). So it begs the question: Why do so many people have gut health disorders?

People with inflammatory bowel disease often suffer pain, cramping, diarrhea, constipation, bleeding stools, fatigue, and weight loss. When a person has a "flare," it can be much more severe and include signs of infection such as fever, chills, and vomiting.

Though people rarely die from IBD, they can die from complications of the disease, such as septic shock from an uncontrolled infection. Though I never experienced this myself, I later had a client who nearly died from this exact scenario. It does happen. A more likely occurrence, however, is a bowel resection or removal of the colon entirely. It is common for doctors to recommend removing the colon and replacing it with a J-pouch for those with severe cases. This often results in improvement of symptoms, but not always in progress in health because the digestive system is permanently impaired.

Causes of Inflammatory Bowel Disease

Ulcerative colitis and related gut issues are often referred to as "idiopathic," meaning: doctors have no idea what causes it. According to the Mayo Clinic, it is an immune system malfunction. Diet and stress only aggravate it but do not cause it. What we do know is that it is an inflammation that is localized to the colon. Toxins, bacteria, viruses, irritants, and stress all cause inflammation.

In the last ten years or so, rates of inflammatory bowel disease have increased significantly. According to the Centers for Disease Control, in 2015, 1.3% of US adults were diagnosed with an inflammatory bowel disease. This is a considerable increase from 1999 when the number was just .9% and has been on a sharp incline since 1950.[11] We have more drugs and medical technology than ever before, yet we also have more chronic diseases than ever before, including inflammatory bowel diseases. It begs the question, what was it that changed in 1950 to send the prevalence of inflammatory bowel disease through the roof?

A literature review concluded that some IBD's de novo could result from bowel altering surgeries, transplantation of organs, stem cells, or fecal microbiome. Also, some medications associated with the development of secondary IBD such as immunomodulators, anti-tumor necrosis factor-alpha agents, anti-interleukin agents, interferons, immune-stimulating agents, and checkpoint inhibitors.

Very little research has been done regarding the use of antibiotics and resulting IBD, but I do know of people who had their first flare within a couple of weeks of taking antibiotics. A recent study in 2020 concluded that "Antibiotics use, particularly antibiotics with a greater spectrum of microbial coverage, may be associated with an increased risk of new-onset inflammatory bowel disease (IBD) and its subtypes ulcerative colitis and Crohn's disease." Antibiotic use may double the risk of getting an inflammatory bowel disease.[12]

My doctor never suggested stress as a possible cause of the disease; however, new research explaining the connection to digestive disorders is emerging. One paper explicitly discusses the effects of stress on the body's inflammatory response. It concludes that "both chronic stress and acute stress are associated with alterations in systemic immune and inflammatory function which may have relevance to the pathogenesis of IBD."[1314]

How Stress Affects The Gut

As I mentioned before, I believe more than ever that mental health and gut health are intertwined. The gut-brain connection has been scientifically proven time and time again.

Stress affects the gut in many ways. The gut contains 500 million neurons. Nerves run from the gut to the brain and messages are sent in both directions. One of the most important nerves is the vagus nerve, which is a cranial nerve and innervates (or runs through) most of the digestive organs. Because the nervous system is connected to the gut, mental health can impair gut dysfunction (and gut dysfunction can also impair mental health).

When the body is in a stressed state, digestive functions are impaired. Instead, it becomes focused on preparing itself to flee or fight. The digestive juices are not necessary for survival and are reduced. This is the sympathetic state of the nervous system, better known as "fight or flight". Humans are hard-wired to have a physical response to danger. Even though the typical daily stressors we humans usually encounter are not dangerous, the body does not know the difference - it is still in the stressed or sympathetic state, and the body responds in the same way.

When the body feels threatened a few distinct things happen in the body. The amygdala (a part of the brain is associated with fear and emotion) sends a distress signal to the hypothalamus that impulses are needed. The adrenal glands secrete adrenaline and cortisol into the bloodstream which creates a cascade of physical reactions. The heart rate goes up, pupils dilate, perspiration increases, muscles become dilated to quickly use glucose to mobilize the body, we become more alert and digestion slows or stops altogether. This is easily overcome when the stressor goes away and we return to the parasympathetic state, but oftentimes we stay in the stressed state because life's stressors are constant.

Can you think of a day that goes by that you don't have a concern about your finances, family, relationships, career, or the state of the world? The fight or flight state is also stimulated by the environment, toxins, and even the way we eat. Most of us live in a stressed state in the modern world and it has simply become our norm. Unfortunately, this is a daily occurrence for many people, as opposed to the unusual danger one might encounter thousands of years ago. In healing, we can oppose this response by turning on the parasympathetic nervous system, but most of us don't have the wherewithal to practice doing so. Especially amidst life's traumas.

The traumas I had as a kid and then as an adult, were affecting my state of health. It was possible that the stress in my life caused gut damage and that the gut damage was exacerbating the anxiety and depression. It all just felt much too big for me to handle independently.

I finally decided it was time to deal with my shit. I made a few calls to potential therapists. One asked me point blank if I had had sexual abuse as a child. I said yes. She asked at what age. The first time I was about six years old, I told her. She said, "I think you are going to need many years of counseling." I immediately hung up on her. Those were things I never discussed with anyone. Ever. It made me uncomfortable to think or talk about any of it. I felt that it would make others uncomfortable too. We aren't responsible for others' feelings, though, are we? Eventually, I called a few more to address my issues and maybe heal my illness. I found a lady, who didn't make me feel like I would vomit over the phone. I was willing to open that door and see what would happen. It was the best decision I ever made.

I would go and see Dr. Smith every week for years. Some weeks were more challenging than others, and I would go twice. She was not easy on me. The first few visits, I didn't like her at all. She seemed like a hard ass. She held the proverbial mirror in front of my face and made me look at my life, and I didn't like that.

She taught me that sometimes things happen in life without reason, and we just have to stop asking "why" and move on. She taught me that guilt can destroy your life and that we do act on information gathered during our childhoods, especially in our relationships.

She helped me sift through the feelings of abandonment when I was a child, the betrayal and fear of men, and the ability to choose our thoughts and actions to help get through it all. Dr. Smith helped me through my divorce and a subsequent toxic relationship. She saw the broken child in me and how I had been letting that hurt little girl affect the woman I am today.

There is so much to learn from self-exploration. We do things that sabotage our lives without even knowing it. I had jumped into a marriage at a young age before I ever really knew what I wanted in life. I chose toxic people that matched my toxic father and often sold myself short on what I believed I deserved in life. I also internalized every emotion, and it ended up manifesting in my gut. Eventually, I recognized that with every bump in the road, my symptoms would worsen. With more emotional upheaval came more blood. It made me learn and recognize the importance of emotional health, and that mine would always take a little effort. And that is ok.

You can't change the past, but you can learn from it and learn to use new coping skills to make it better. She was one of the most helpful and influential people in my life. I did end up going to counseling for years, as the lady I hung up on suggested. It was the most beautiful experience, though, and if Dr. Smith didn't retire, I would still be going today. It was an essential step in my healing, and I am always aware that my mental state is directly tied to my gut health.

Not Giving Up

I was never one to accept defeat. I would find a way, whatever it was. Challenges never deterred me in the past. I had moved to Vegas by myself at 18, bought my first house at 19, and put myself through college with no outside help. I pulled through near-death experiences and even had my babies at home with no drugs. I had done hard things before and had no doubt I could handle this. I read stories of others who had the disease and found something to try that others had used. There was hope, and I would not give up without finding a solution. I knew there were better options than drugs and surgery.

I would spend the next 6 years experimenting with every diet and remedy possible. I had a new obsession, and it was healing this illness with some sort of diet or natural remedy.

I believed it was possible, and that if I could just find the right combination soon enough, I would be ok.

There seemed to be something within the combination of stress and irritants that come up for people with IBD, so identifying irritants was the path I was going down.

---

[10] https://www.drugs.com/sfx/lialda-side-effects.html

[11] www.cdc.gov

[12] https://www.sciencedaily.com/releases/2020/08/200817191743.htm

[13] https://www.ncbi.nlm.nih.gov/pmc/articles/PMC1774724/

[14] Mawdsley JE, Rampton DS. *Psychological stress in IBD: new insights into pathogenic and therapeutic implications. Gut. 2005*;54(10):1481-1491. doi:10.1136/gut.2005.064261

FOUR: SEARCHING FOR AN ANSWER THROUGH FOOD

If you have ever really looked for a diet, you will find thousands out there. In fact, a 2020 poll found that the average person tries 126 different diets in their lifetime.[15]

Most are for weight loss, but there are also many related to the gut and healing of others disorders as well. I found some specific to Crohn's and colitis in my search for answers. One at a time, I would give each plan a try. Some I would follow for weeks and some for many months. I would adhere strictly to the recommendations and pray for results.

Time after time, I would try a diet and perhaps see a slight change, but inevitably the symptoms would come right back. In the process, I learned a lot about food that most people never do. This was partly due to my incessant research, but mostly from my personal experience.

There is so much information available regarding diets. About 5 million diet books are sold every year in the United States alone. There are countless different diets, and one has to do tremendous research to figure out which one might apply to their needs. Most target weight loss, but there are still thousands that are intended to cure any number of ailments.

Strangely, diets specific to inflammatory bowel or gut health in general are relatively limited. Furthermore, there is no diet that works for everyone, you just have to learn for yourself. I don't regret the process - it was a path of discovery and learning that eventually brought me my answers, and helped me to understand what people are dealing with - and how to best help them. It would eventually help both myself and my clients.

The first plan I tried was a low glycemic diet. The premise with low glycemic foods is that they will balance the blood sugar, resulting in lowered cortisol and lowered inflammation. It was also very effective for weight loss. I had helped to develop a weight loss program for a company I consulted for, and thousands of people were losing weight, coming off blood pressure and cholesterol medications, it was highly effective for many people. The diet included animal protein, lots of low-carb veggies such as broccoli and spinach, and fruit. It was very much like keto before keto was a thing and I still use it today for many clients due to the wide variety of food available and it is not too strict.

I felt lighter on this plan, easily maintained my body weight and my energy was good. Unfortunately, the colon problems would come and go. Every day was different, and the longest I would go without bleeding was just a couple of days, then it would reliably return. It wasn't the answer, but I was learning that food DID affect me and did make a difference. Was it one of the veggies I was eating that showed promise? I ate a lot of variety each day, so pinpointing anything was going to be difficult. I tried eliminating eggs one week, strawberries the next. Nothing really changed.

I returned to the raw vegan diet, getting out my dehydrators, sprouted chickpea hummus, and flaxseed crackers. This diet is essentially made of fruits, vegetables, nuts and seeds. Nothing was heated over 105 degrees to prevent damaging the food's natural enzymes. I was actually kind of excited to try raw veganism again because it seemed very labor-intensive and that must be good for something! Every day took hours of prepping with all the washing, chopping, soaking, and sprouting of foods. Food prep was my part-time job, but I was willing to do anything so I did.

In my previous years as a vegan, I ate a lot of nuts and seeds. I made smoothies, crackers, nut butter, cashew milk, and I didn't have bleeding stools. Perhaps this time it would work! Within days I had horrendous bloating, pain, and bleeding stools; veganism was an assault to my gut. I had read about others who had success on vegan and plant-based diets, so I shifted to eating cooked vegan foods such as beans and vegetables. Still, my symptoms raged on. There was no sign of improvement, only an undeniable worsening from veganism. I had to acknowledge that veganism in any form, was not the answer for me.

Next up was the macrobiotic diet, which consisted of grains, legumes, root vegetables, and seaweed. This diet originated in Japan and has been adopted by other countries as an anticancer and anti-inflammatory diet. The macrobiotic approach considers meat to be toxic and was strictly forbidden on this plan as it was considered to be the worst possible food for the colon because it is considered acidic. The macrobiotic approach strives for pH balance, and adding more alkaline foods was touted as the way to do that.

I took this to be a spin-off of the vegan diet, although this one focuses on including a lot of grains that are specifically prepared to remove phytates. This made good sense since phytates do inhibit the absorption of nutrients and also can irritate the gut. Again, I followed the diet to the letter. I soaked every grain, prepared all foods as directed, and waited. I saw no changes in my symptoms, but started to gain weight and feel sluggish. Another fail. Moving away from animal proteins didn't improve my condition, and didn't make me feel good in general.

I reviewed where I had been so far and what had produced the best results for me. At that point, it was clear that I did best on the low glycemic program I had given many clients for weight loss. Plant-based diets were not the answer for me, and eating some protein had me feeling my best. All I could do was listen to my body and move in that direction. I continued to research diets that included animal protein but were sensitive to gut issues.

One dietary approach that is often used for autoimmune diseases is the Autoimmune Protocol (AIP) diet plan. The goal of this plan is to reduce foods that cause inflammation by eliminating those that irritate the gut or cause gut permeability. The AIP completely avoids grains, legumes, nuts, seeds, nightshade vegetables, eggs, and dairy.

Although not foods, the Autoimmune Protocol also eliminates other things that may contribute to gut inflammation such as alcohol, coffee, oils and food additives as well as anti inflammatory drugs like NSAIDS. I did follow this protocol for several months and found that it did reduce the severity of my symptoms somewhat, though never resolved them completely. This diet did still include many vegetables such as leafy greens and cruciferous vegetables, which may have still been too much for my gut to handle with ulcerative colitis.

Another diet that was touted as the best for my condition was the Specific Carbohydrate Diet. The SCD was an elimination diet of sorts, strictly prohibiting grains in any form. Instead, it focused on eating cheese, eggs, fruits, and vegetables. This sounded reasonable enough, and I had already learned enough negative things about grains. I had read of others who had success with taming inflammatory bowel conditions using the SCD so it definitely made the list of possibilities.

After starting the diet, I would get reduced symptoms for a couple of weeks; then, bleeding would return. The diet includes meat, cheese, fruits, most vegetables, nuts, and legumes. Essentially, this diet promotes whole foods and eliminates most processed grains. It has been used for Crohn's disease and some people do get good results from following it. I gave this plan a couple of months, following religiously, to no avail. I continued to have bleeding stools and stomach cramps almost daily.

In 2017, I tried the ketogenic diet because it was said to produce ketones in the body, and be anti-inflammatory. The ketogenic diet is high fat, moderate protein and very low carbohydrate. The premise is that the body makes ketones when glucose is not available and one of those ketones, beta hydroxybutyrate, is considered highly anti-inflammatory.

Since colitis is an inflammation of the gut lining, I thought this made a lot of sense. Keto is wildly popular because it produces rapid weight loss in some people (because the high fat diets reduce appetite so people eat less calories) and also because the lack of carbohydrates increase adrenaline which increases lipolysis, or fat burning. In addition, people lose a lot of water due to the drop in insulin so they lose weight rapidly, both water and body fat.

Even though this was not the reason I was interested in it, there has been a tremendous amount of support from the medical fields and entire movements based on the ketogenic diet. In researching the keto diet I looked to Stephen Phinney and Jeff Volek, two of the pioneers and researchers in the field of low carb diets. Their first book, *The Art and Science of Low Carb Living*, was a good manual for learning the science behind low carb diets and how to use them. My ketogenic diet consisted mostly of fatty chicken, salmon and vegetables. After a few months I added in keto baked goods, fat bombs, and treats made of peanut butter and butter. Looking back I didn't know that the vegetables I ate were gut irritant and the almond breads and treats were loaded with lectins and oxalates. That was a very "fun" diet but didn't fix the issue. I continued to bleed, but I had lowered energy and started gaining weight on top of that.

When you feel lousy every day you become desperate to find answers, I was willing to try anything. I knew diet was related to colitis because when I changed my diet, my gut would respond. So there had to be a connection between what I was eating and my symptoms. Even though my doctor told me that it didn't matter what I ate, I knew better than this. That made no sense at all, and I had little trust in medical doctors from all I had seen.

Along with the various diets, I tried probiotics, nutraceuticals, herbal supplements, vitamins, and even bee venom from Australia. I spent thousands of dollars over the years on every pill, potion, and promise of better gut health. Though at times my symptoms seemed lessened, they just would not completely cease. I would sometimes see a slight improvement for a few days, but it never lasted.

At one point, I came across a product intended to heal the gut lining by healing the tight junctions of the lining that was destroyed by glyphosate, the chemical in seed and in the pesticide *Roundup*. Although it didn't give me any relief while researching plants with high amounts of chemicals, I came across the book by Dr. Gundry, *The Plant Paradox*. This book describes how lectins naturally occur in many plant foods, which are detrimental to the gut. This concept made sense to me because after retrying the vegan diet with terrible results; it occurred to me that I had been eating a diet very high in lectins. I followed Dr. Gundry's diet for a couple of months. I saw improvement, but the disease hung on. I was getting somewhere, though, and a cure was within reach.

YouTube is a great place to find information if you can sift through the nonsense. The best part of YouTube is; the videos of the average Jane or Joe talking about their experience with X,Y or Z. I was following keto accounts for tips and recipes and came across what I considered a radical and absurd diet, the carnivore diet. The face of this diet was Dr. Shawn Baker. Dr. Baker is an osteopathic surgeon that stands at 6'6, 230 lbs of what appeared to be pure muscle. He is also a World Champion athlete in rowing. His secret weapon? He ate nothing but meat and trained like a beast.

Dr. Baker shared his experience as a physician and surgeon with patients dramatically improving their joint problems by following this diet. He posted pictures and videos on social media of all the people who followed the carnivore diet and healed some illnesses. People eating the only meat diet were healing joints, skin problems and even mental health disorders. They would lose weight, gain muscle and claim to feel better than they ever have in their life. Many people had cured autoimmune diseases of all sorts, and this got my attention.

My initial thought was, this is ridiculous. I watched all of Shawn's videos, following closely for months to make sense of what he was saying. His website was filled with stories of healing using the diet, hundreds of them. Eventually I found one person with a story like mine who had used the carnivore diet to heal his ulcerative colitis. I was skeptical but kept digging. If one person could do it, then it was at least a slim possibility.

The carnivore world is ripe with dogma, just as any diet culture. This comes with the territory when talking about diets, as many people vehemently defend their diet as strongly as they do their religion. Ultimately you have to do what works for you, and it doesn't work for everyone. Some people talked about endless diarrhea, some of weight gain, some of low energy. I had heard some negative comments from women who had lost their periods, and some that had headaches and lethargy that was nearly debilitating. It wasn't all positive, but the majority of the personal accounts I had read, however, were all about healing. People were eating nothing but meat and healing diseases and ailments that they had been suffering from, sometimes for their entire lives.

[15] https://www.independent.co.uk/life-style/diet-weight-loss-food-unhealthy-eating-habits-a9274676.html

FIVE: FINALLY HEALING

The diet that I was embarking on was restrictive because it removes all possible irritants, allowing the gut to heal. Like many people who try out a special diet, I fumbled a lot in the beginning. The carnivore diet is defined differently by different people, but I viewed it as a diet devoid of plants.

Plants, I learned, contained many things that are very bad for your gut and overall health. For example, I never realized that the fiber in most leafy greens, cellulose, is not digested by the human stomach. It turns out that animals who eat grasses and leaves have a rumen or second stomach in which they can break down the cellulose and absorb the nutrients from it. Humans do not have this capability, so eating cellulose can cause irritation to the gut and cause an increase in endotoxins in the bowel. Kale was a huge part of my diet when I was vegan, in fact, I would eat it at least 3-4 days per week, and oftentimes daily. The leafy greens I was so intentional about eating were wiped off the list of food options.

Some vegetables also contain lectins, which cause inflammation and irritation to the gut lining. Lectins are found in most plants but are highest in legumes and grains, which are a staple in vegan and plant-based diets. They are thought to be naturally occurring in plants to prevent predators such as insects or animals from eating them. For humans, they cause inflammation and irritation of the gut. I didn't mind excluding legumes and grains because I always felt bloated from eating them, and it was amazing how much better my stomach felt once I did.

The broccoli and cauliflower I used to eat on most days were also eliminated. Not only do they contain lectins and fiber, but undercooked cruciferous vegetables also contain goitrogens (explained in the table below) that can harm the thyroid. If you think about it, it's not very "natural" to eat plants that are primarily grown in huge agriculture farms. I tried growing broccoli myself before; it takes a lot of space to cultivate the amount of broccoli that I was eating. One plant would yield about 1 cup of broccoli. I would eat at least 5-6 cups of broccoli per week when I was vegan. Growing enough to support my habit would only be possible by the average person. Also, where in nature have you ever seen broccoli or cauliflower growing in nature?

Sadly, I learned that the nuts and seeds that tasted so good were high in oxalates and phytic acid and could also be very irritating to the gut. I had become in the habit of making all sorts of paleo cookies and breads with almond flour, not knowing that these seemingly healthy treats could have been worsening my condition. I had been drinking almond milk for years, and I had learned that carrageenan, a common emulsifier, was very annoying to the gut and even caused chronic inflammation.

The "Healthy" Foods I Gave Up To Heal Myself

The diet that I was embarking on was restrictive because it removes all possible irritants, allowing the gut to heal. Like many people who try out a special diet, I fumbled a lot in the beginning. The carnivore diet is defined differently by different people, but I viewed it as a diet devoid of plants.

Plants, I learned, contained many things that are very bad for your gut and overall health. For example, I never realized that the fiber in most leafy greens, cellulose, is not digested by the human stomach. It turns out that animals who eat grasses and leaves have a rumen or second stomach in which they can break down the cellulose and absorb the nutrients from it. Humans do not have this capability, so eating cellulose can cause irritation to the gut and cause an increase in endotoxins in the bowel. Kale was a huge part of my diet when I was vegan, in fact, I would eat it at least 3-4 days per week, and oftentimes daily. The leafy greens I was so intentional about eating were wiped off the list of food options.

Some vegetables also contain lectins, which cause inflammation and irritation to the gut lining. Lectins are found in most plants but are highest in legumes and grains, which are a staple in vegan and plant-based diets. They are thought to be naturally occurring in plants to prevent predators such as insects or animals from eating them. For humans, they cause inflammation and irritation of the gut. I didn't mind excluding legumes and grains because I always felt bloated from eating them, and it was amazing how much better my stomach felt once I did.

The broccoli and cauliflower I used to eat on most days were also eliminated. Not only do they contain lectins and fiber, but undercooked cruciferous vegetables also contain goitrogens that can harm the thyroid. If you think about it, it's not very "natural" to eat plants that are primarily grown in huge agriculture farms. I tried growing broccoli myself before; it takes a lot of space to cultivate the amount of broccoli that I was eating. One plant would yield about 1 cup of broccoli. I would eat at least 5-6 cups of broccoli per week when I was vegan. Growing enough to support my habit would only be possible by the average person. Also, where in nature have you ever seen broccoli or cauliflower growing in nature?

Sadly, I learned that the nuts and seeds that tasted so good were high in oxalates and phytic acid and could also be very irritating to the gut. I had become in the habit of making all sorts of paleo cookies and breads with almond flour, not knowing that these seemingly healthy treats could have been worsening my condition. I had been drinking almond milk for years, and I had learned that carrageenan, a common emulsifier, was very annoying to the gut and even caused chronic inflammation.

Antinutrients	Food Sources	Clinical Implications
Lectins	Legumes, cereal grains, seeds, nuts. Fruits and vegetables	Altered gut function, inflammation
Oxalates	Rhubarb, chard, sorrel, beet greens, nuts, legumes, cereal grains, sweet potatoes and potatoes.	May increase calcium kidney stone formation.
Phytates	Legumes, grains, amaranth, quinoa and millet	May inhibit absorption of iron and calcium.
Goitrogens	Kale, Brussels sprouts, broccoli, cabbage, millet	Hypothyroidism and/or goiter. Inhibit iodine uptake
Phytoestrogens	Soy products, flaxseeds, nuts, fruits and vegetables	Endocrine disruption, increased risk of estrogen-sensitive cancers
Tannins	Tea, cacao, grapes, berries, apples, stone fruits, beans, whole grains	Inhibit iron absorption, negatively impact iron stores

TABLE 1[16]

All of this means nuts and seeds are probably not something someone with an inflamed colon should be consuming. Nuts and seeds also contain phytic acid which can irritate the gastrointestinal tract causing stomach pains and minerals such as calcium, magnesium, iron, and zinc from being absorbed during digestion. Those minerals are critical to metabolism and thyroid function, which when impaired can lead to inflammatory diseases including inflammatory bowel disease.

One of the most frustrating things to see is the promotion of almond, cashew, and other nuts and seeds made into a milk substitute. Not only do they contain phytic acid and oftentimes gums or thickeners that can irritate the gut but they also contain polyunsaturated fats which can oxidize in the body and also impair thyroid function. In short, nuts and seeds in all formats can do harm to your gut and thyroid.

We have become accustomed to fruits and vegetables being the cornerstone of a healthy diet. Who determined that we should eat foods that are only mass-produced through large-scale agriculture?

We have been taught since we were kids to eat our veggies, so to think that they could be causing us harm is a very different way of thinking. The hardest part of the carnivore diet was not actually the diet but letting go of the lifetime of messaging that has been pre-programmed into our brains about nutrition.

We have been told that meat is unhealthy, that saturated fat will kill you, and that your diet should consist mostly of grains, legumes, veggies, and fruit. When we start to understand that vegetables were never available to humans as they are today, we also have to accept that they may never have been intended for us to eat.

Seed Oils, One of The Most Dangerous Foods

One of the most important things I learned during my healing journey was that oils that come from seeds are one of the most toxic things to the human body. These are also referred to as industrial oils, and can include canola oil, grapeseed oil, corn oil, soybean oil, generic vegetable oil, walnut oil, cottonseed oil, sesame oil, peanut oil, hemp oil, margarine, and flaxseed oil. Fish oil, although touted as an anti-inflammatory Omega 3 fatty acid, is also a polyunsaturated fatty acid and easily oxidizes, especially the capsules sold in health food stores.

Animal foods also contain polyunsaturated fatty acids. Cows and chickens fed corn and soy have polyunsaturated fatty acids in their tissues and byproducts such as eggs. The canola oil that replaced the saturated fats we were told would kill us actually are some of the most toxic "foods" to the human body.

Seed oils, or polyunsaturated fatty acids, are not intended for the human body and are in fact a waste by-product of the grain and seed industry that is intended to feed livestock. For this reason I always choose pasture-raised, grass fed beef, pork, chicken and lamb. Even some farm-raised fish are fed corn and soy and will have elevated polyunsaturated fatty acids content, so wild-caught fish and seafood is a safer choice. Even the so-called "healthy" nuts and seeds promoted as healthy snacking are rich sources of polyunsaturated fatty acids and are best avoided.

Polyunsaturated fatty acids (also referred to as PUFAs) are highly toxic to the body because they are unstable and go rancid very quickly. Once these fats are oxidized they create high levels of free radicals that cause aging and damage to the tissues, intestines and organs. They can affect the thyroid and the entire metabolic system.

I recall my mother making what she considered to be very healthy cookies for us that were made with canola oil, and you can still find it on health food store shelves in abundance. In fact, salad dressings, which are promoted as a part of healthy salad eating diets, almost always include some if not all of their base ingredients as PUFA oil, namely soy oil.[17]

By this point, you might begin to wonder, what *is* safe to eat? This is why the carnivore diet can be so effective, but it is also what makes it restrictive and that can be a challenge for many people. Part of finding what foods irritate you is eliminating the choices. When you narrow it down to only animal foods, the least irritating of all foods, it becomes easier to identify problems. Early on, I still ate a spoonful of peanut butter, chewed gum, and drank alcohol on occasion. I learned that all of those things could deter the healing of your gut, even in small amounts. It was a whole new concept, not eating plants.

I had focused on fruits and vegetables most of my life; this was how I thought you got your nutrients as a human. It turns out you don't; humans just don't have the mechanisms needed to break down and absorb many of the nutrients found in plants. However, animals do and their bodies can store the nutrients we need. When we eat animal-based diets we can obtain all of the nutrients needed to stay healthy, with little to no irritation on our digestive system.

*

But Aren't Plant-Based Diets The Healthiest Choice?

Plant-based diets are hailed as the healthiest diet for preventing disease and managing weight. I have learned that this simply is not the case. I did all of the research in my early days of veganism and you can certainly find compelling evidence to support it. You can also find the opposite, and I have come to the realization in both my personal life and professional career in Public Health, that just because a study is published describing the benefits of something, does not make it true.

There are many research studies that are flawed due to the way they are conducted or through biases. Many nutrition studies are conducted via epidemiology, which requires participants to answer a long line of questions about their dietary habits. They can be obscure and difficult to answer - also, people are not always truthful. Other studies are funded by organizations that stand to benefit financially from certain results, and even more are designed with researchers who are even paid to prove a certain point. Statistics can easily be manipulated, and they are. Unfortunately, we can not always trust science.

Plant-based diets are considered healthy because they are high in fiber, low in saturated fats, and high in vitamins and minerals. I would agree there are some benefits to fruits and vegetables such as minerals, fiber for the microbiome, and glucose to fuel the body, however, agriculture has created foods that have become trendy but problematic for our guts.

It turns out that inflamed intestines really don't appreciate more fiber in the diet. What most people aren't told is that fiber can be highly irritating to the gut, especially if it is already inflamed. One of the worst pieces of advice for someone with inflammatory bowel disease is to eat more fiber.

Humans do not possess the digestive capabilities to break down insoluble fiber. It can get stuck in the intestines and ferment, and even cause Small Intestinal Bacterial Overgrowth (SIBO) which can be very difficult to get rid of. Some fibers such as cellulose are common in the "health food" scene such as kale salads and other salads, however, humans just aren't capable of breaking down this fiber, so it ultimately causes a lot of inflammation and irritation in the colon, as well as ferments and causes endotoxins to build up in the gut.

So why are we told to eat fiber? In my humble opinion, like most things, it comes down to money. Much of the nutrition research conducted is to demonstrate a need for a product, such as a fiber supplement. Research can easily be biased or manipulated to shine a positive light on a product to increase sales or demonstrate need.

Humans never needed such things in the past, and they certainly didn't eat mass quantities of fiber like the Food and Drug Administration would like you to believe. Just take a look at your favorite natural landscape. When was the last time you saw broccoli or cauliflower growing along your hiking path? How about some kale? Do you know how many beans you would have to collect to have a bowl of hummus? Some of these health foods are just unrealistic when you put them in the context of what nature provides to us humans, and that is how we have to think.

Other irritating foods that are eliminated on the carnivore diet were lectins that are found in legumes, nuts, seeds, and some vegetables. Broccoli, for example, was a major staple in my diet along with all other cruciferous veggies such as cauliflower, cabbage, and loads of kale. I remember making huge green smoothies with almond milk (lectins) and kale (cellulose and goitrogens) and never figured it was the reason I felt so bloated.

I would later learn that these foods not only tore up my stomach but also contain goitrogens, which can negatively affect the thyroid by suppressing the release of thyroid hormones. I was eating most of these raw because I wasn't aware of goitrogens or that cooking them will greatly reduce the goitrogen content.

Another concern about eating a lot of vegetables is glyphosate exposure. Glyphosate is a chemical within the seed of many vegetable crops that inhibits fungal or insect damage. In an article by U.S. Right To Know, it is considered the most widely used herbicide and has been classified as a probable human carcinogen by the World Health Organization.[18]

Unfortunately, it has also been very destructive to the human gut, as it inflames the intestinal lining and can lead to intestinal permeability or leaky gut. One study published in *Interdisciplinary Toxicology* in 2013 proposed that the chemical may be the cause of the rise in celiac disease, a gut health disease that causes gluten intolerance specifically.[19]

Leaky gut occurs when inflammation in the gut lining causes a loosening of the tight junctions, allowing materials in the digestive tract to pass through the tiny openings into the bloodstream, which the body sees as invaders in the blood and may launch an attack against them. Many people with various autoimmune diseases improve once they limit gut irritants in their diet, which is a good hint that the gut inflammation goes down and things can go back to normal, as it did with me.

Lies and Profit Over Meat and Fats

In her incredible book, *The Big Fat Surprise*, Nina Teicholz exposes the truth about the health of people eating animal foods and the lies made about meats and saturated fats initiated by Ancel Keys in the 1950's. He proposed that saturated fats from beef, eggs, milk and cheese were the cause of the rising levels of heart disease. He suggested a low-fat diet as the healthiest diet and least likely to cause heart disease.This was the turning point in America, where animal fats became demonized and unsaturated fats became the "healthy" fats even though there was no research to prove it. He became known as "Mr. Cholesterol" as he demonized it and recommended dietary fats comprise just 15% of the American diet.

Keys along with the American Heart Association and the National Institutes of Health shifted the American diet to monopolize the attention and direction of Americans and how they should be eating. Their efforts were funded by Procter & Gamble, the world's largest consumer goods manufacturer who raised millions of dollars to fund the campaigns on nutrition. In 1948, P&G donated millions to the American Heart Association who provided guidance on the healthiest diets to prevent heart disease. Their messaging was simple: eat less meat and fat and more grains in order to reduce heart disease. Procter & Gamble is one of the largest producers of the unsaturated fats from corn and soy that were being pushed as the safe and healthy fat. Lard that was a longtime cooking fat was now replaced with Crisco, and the marketing was targeted to the lady of the house as the one in charge of feeding and cooking for their family. They were told it was the healthier and cheaper substitute for lard, and that the most progressive and smartest women were transitioning from lard to Crisco.

Seed oils originated as a by-product of the cotton industry. Cotton was grown for fabrics but had a large portion of waste in the form of seed. Cotton seed was then pressed for its oil, and after much processing and deodorization becomes a clear unsaturated fat that can be used for various things including personal care products and candles, but ultimately made its debut as a "healthy" alternative to lard for use in cooking and baking after the inception of chemical processing called hydrogenation which made a liquid oil solid in order to replicate lard.

Its safety or long term use results were never tested, but it brought huge products to what would otherwise be a waste product. Later on, soybean would take its place. It was cheaper to grow and yielded more materials to work with. From the soybean they could make livestock feed, soybean oil and industrial uses such as lubricants and paint. There was no evidence that soy was safe and healthy, yet it was a profitable crop so more products needed to be made and sold from it.

Since the soybean has a high protein content, it was first used as a livestock feed, but soon would be shifted to be marketed and sold to us lucky Americans. Soy formula was the new healthy alternative to breast milk, and eventually tofu was the healthy alternative to meat. It just so happens that soybean is an inexpensive crop to produce, but can yield billions of dollars when food manufacturers adopt it as a staple ingredient in their products. Soybean oil and soy derivatives continue to be sold as ingredients in the manufacturing of thousands of foods, even those sold in natural food stores. You can go into any health food or regular grocery store today and nearly any packaged food on the shelf will have some derivative of soy as an ingredient.

Politics Over Health

Who determines what is healthy? Where are these guidelines coming from?

The U.S. Department of Health and Human Services (HHS) and the U.S. Department of Agriculture (USDA) jointly publishes the Dietary Guidelines for Americans every 5 years. These recommendations are biased because those that profit from the recommendation of certain foods (grains, legumes and seed oils) are the ones in charge of making the dietary guidelines for Americans.

There is a very clear conflict of interest in the powers that control the food supply and who designs the suggested foods for all of our schools, hospitals, government and medical establishments to recommend. On the HHS website, they state that their recommendations are based on scientific research. Based on what we know about research, it can report anything they want it to report. Research can be highly biased and manipulated and often reflects outcomes that benefit those that fund the research.

In addition, the USDA's primary stakeholders are major food producers and manufacturers, who will recommend their products be included as part of nutritional guidelines. Either way, there is a large amount of money at stake that is won or lost by big agriculture as a result of their guidelines to Americans, so you can be sure they will do anything to influence the recommendations in favor of their commercial products.

Why are grains and legumes promoted over grass-fed meat and dairy? Profit!

Grass-fed meats and dairy are not profitable to big agriculture and quite honestly, not to big pharma either. Just imagine all of the drugs that are given to those with digestive disorders that would be no longer needed if each of those individuals ate whole food diets that healed their disease.

Ultimately, to heal my health, I learned to eat meat and animal products again while eliminating most of the foods I had always believed to be healthy. I realized very quickly that just because it was plant food didn't mean I should eat it. Everything I was doing was completely backwards from everything I learned from my personal studies, but also from my education in public health.

In Public Health, the FDA guidelines are followed by every facet of the medical model and continue to recommend little to no animal proteins and high amounts of plants and grains. The common rhetoric of low saturated fat in favor of unsaturated fats and less meat in favor of more grains and legumes was what we were taught to teach others. I was learning that this was a very flawed approach, and worst of all was driven by profit over health.

Why Physicians Don't Offer More Help With Diets

You may be thinking that while these dietary recommendations are given to the average American, something different is recommended for people with digestive diseases.

Not so.

Although I believe most doctors mean well, they simply do not have the training or tools to help people with their nutrition because their medical programs do not include what is needed for them to learn it. Those that will choose to add additional training on nutrition beyond medical school may be more skilled in advising their patients in the area of nutrition.

Unfortunately, very little nutrition advice was offered to me by my gastroenterologist. According to the American Gastroenterological Association, adequate nutrition education and training is lacking among physicians, even those in the gastroenterology field. According to the AGA there have been several studies demonstrating this deficiency.

As of 2010, U.S. medical schools offer less than 20 hours of nutrition education within a four year medical school program.[20]

A 2014 study examined 32 Canadian gastroenterology fellows and performed a needs assessment as well as a 40-question multiple choice examination. The majority of fellows did not receive nutrition education in medical school and their perceived knowledge was lowest with respect to obesity and macronutrient/micronutrient requirements.[2122]

According to a 2015 report in the Journal of Biomedical Education, only 29 percent of U.S. medical schools offer medical students the recommended 25 hours of nutrition education.[23]

So it is no surprise that medical school graduates in a 2016 study only answered 52% of their nutrition questions correctly when tested prior to their residency program.[24]

In our society, we have a strong sense of authoritarianism. People have been indoctrinated to follow the advice of someone in a position of authority such as a physician or government body. The unfortunate thing is that government recommendations are heavily influenced by special interests - and physicians typically don't have the knowledge base.

Our dietary guidelines include foods that not only profit the supplier, but also hurt the consumer. Grains and legumes are very well known gut irritants, though they work slowly to disintegrate health. People often consume these foods for years before realizing they have problems with their health, then have trouble pinpointing what could be the problem.

Then you have people that do not follow the dietary guidelines but instead follow what has come to be known as the Standard American Diet, which is rife with processed foods.

The Dietary Guidelines for Americans for 2020-2025 recommends 6oz per day of grains, divided equally between refined and whole grains. Knowing that grains can cause inflammation due to their lectins and glyphosate, this small amount eaten daily is enough to cause significant irritation in some individuals.

In addition, grains hold the LEAST amount of vitamins and minerals of all the other foods with the exception of dietary fats, so why do they make the largest proportion of dietary recommendations? We certainly need carbohydrates, but those can be obtained adequately through fruit and vegetable consumption. We also know that Americans will certainly take it upon themselves to include this higher proportion of grains, so the likelihood of it making up an even higher portion of the diet is highly possible.

According to Tufts University, as of 2019 Americans are eating 42% of their calories from refined carbohydrates which may be due to access to foods that are highly marketed such as pizzas, chips and sandwiches.[25]

Similarly, other foods that are deemed healthy, such as leafy greens, legumes and starchy vegetables are included in the amounts of 2 ½ cups per day. These foods are also very problematic for those with compromised digestion and may cause future problems for those that don't, due to the high amounts of cellulose, goitrogens and lectins found in nearly all of those foods.

When digestion is compromised and foods are not digested properly, they can remain in the intestines for longer periods of time which breed endotoxin bacteria that causes inflammation in the gut lining.[26]

Healthy US Style Dietary Pattern at 2000 Calorie Level With Daily or Weekly Amounts From Foodgroups

Food Group	Daily Amount From Each Group (vegetable and protein amounts are per week)
Vegetables	
Dark Green Leafy Vegetables	2 ½
Red and Orange Vegetables	5 ½
Beans, Peas, Lentils	1 ½
Starchy Vegetables	1 ½
Other Vegetables	4
Fruits cup/day	2
Grains ounce/day	6
Whole Grains	>3
Refined Grains	<3
Dairy	3
Protein Foods ounce/day	5 ½
Meats ounce / week	26
Seafood ounce / week	8
Nuts, Seeds, Soy Products ounce / week	6
Oils	27
Limit on Calories for Other Uses Cal/day	240
Limit on Calories for Other Uses %/day	12

TABLE 2[27]

When I First Saw Changes By Eliminating "Healthy" Foods

After a few starts and restarts, I finally got into the groove and found my way through the carnivore diet. I had coffee with eggs and bacon for breakfast and often skipped lunch, having a steak or lamb for dinner. Most of my meals were made of ruminant animals. Since they have a rumen or second stomach, they can digest plant fibers that we humans cannot. As a result, they absorb all of the nutrients, and their bodies become a great source of nutrients to us humans.

Since I was not eating any carbohydrates, I would be eating a large proportion of fat to protein, and that kept me extremely satiated. It is not uncommon for people on the carnivore diet to eat just two or even one meal per day. This has some downsides to it, but in terms of healing the gut, having less food going through the body does give the intestines a break and allows them time to heal.

Within days of limiting myself to meat, fish, chicken, eggs and bacon I found myself having much less bloating. My stomach quickly flattened out and the discomfort that I had become accustomed to suddenly vanished. Not only did my bloating disappear, but fat from my abdominal region, which was not a lot previously, also disappeared. I was becoming very lean, and also feeling calmer. My digestion was improving and the bleeding in the stools slowed over the coming week. I did have the notorious diarrhea that comes with the carnivore diet, but it only lasted a couple of weeks and was a huge trade up from how I was feeling before.

I was inspired and hopeful with the changes. Just like in the past with previous diets, I was dedicated. I followed the plan strictly, and saw small changes and improvements every day. It was not a struggle, but I was not going to cheat in the slightest. It isn't hard to follow a diet of steaks, juicy hamburgers, crabby legs and lobster. I enjoyed the food and I was propelled by optimism to keep going forward. There was improvement enough to believe it just might work, and I felt terrific. I had zero bloating or discomfort in my stomach, my hair loss stopped and I was feeling lean and strong. Elated with my results, I pressed on.

New Nicole!

Four months into my carnivore experience, something miraculous happened. The bleeding stopped. The last symptom to plague me for years, finally went away. It stayed away for weeks, and the fear in me calmed. I was nervous and waiting for it to return, waiting for the pins and needles I felt in my ribs to flare up. It never came though, and as I write this book for you today, I have not had a single symptom of ulcerative colitis, almost 4 years later.

Some people like to call this "remission", I call it "healing". Later I will tell you why I believe this, since I am now able to eat a variety of food, but this is where the healing began. By taking the steps to remove what my body could no longer deal with (fiber, lectins, emotions) it could finally take a step forward to a life without disease.

For all the years I spent trying to eat as many vegetables as possible, I never would have thought that I would come to my best health by avoiding them. For most people, it is considered the cornerstone of a healthy diet. This information can now be found more easily since the work of many people to debunk the ideas that meat and saturated fats are unhealthy, and that vegetables and plant-based diets are superior is widely available. I have since found plenty of evidence to the contrary as well as my first-hand experience.

In 2018, after one year on the carnivore diet I decided to have my routine lab work done. I found that my thyroid levels had improved from the past where it had required thyroid medication. I had normal cholesterol levels and very good HDL levels. My glucose was a bit high, at 5.6, but I had been eating low carb for quite some time, which I later learned can increase HBA1C.

All the while I followed the diet and saw my disease subside and then vanish, I never stopped getting heat from people. They would warm me that meat would kill me, that I would have a heart attack, or that I would be malnourished without vegetables. None of those things happened. I was strong and lean, had no inflammation that I could tell, my skin looked good and I could physically do all the things I love to do.

The problems that I had as a result of a damaged gut (like poor nutrient absorption, anxiety, joint pain, thyroid problems and poor immunity) all had improved or resolved over the course of two years. On paper I was perfectly healthy, but more importantly, I no longer struggled with the health issues that had plagued me for so many years.

Astonishingly, without any drugs or surgeries, my battle with colitis was over.

Adding Foods Back In

I continued to follow the diet for another year and a half. Eating only animal products for two and a half years didn't kill me, it actually saved my life. However, I was starting to notice that some things were changing. I was having trouble sleeping and the anxiety I had when I was vegan seemed to return. I was beginning to gain weight and my hair was dry and breaking. I had intense cravings for fruit and sweets. Something was off and I knew it.

In December of 2019, I had appendicitis, which led me to spend 3 days in the hospital recovering from appendectomy with intravenous antibiotics. No one knows what causes it and it is somewhat rare to have it as an adult, but I was not eating the foods considered to trigger it, which is nuts and seeds. Between the appendicitis and how I was feeling, I decided I was ready to try changing my diet to see if I would notice an improvement without compromising the seemingly good condition of my gut.

I decided to do labs yet again, this time with a 24 urinalysis to look more at hormones. I felt I had gained some weight without really changing my diet, so I wanted to learn more about what might be causing this. It was also the time Coronavirus had emerged and I was feeling very stressed about what was happening around me. You can never discount the effects of stress.

Nonetheless, the results showed extremely high cortisol and no testosterone. On top of that I had excess estrogen that I was evidently not detoxifying very well. I started to research these and got heavily versed in stress and what causes high cortisol. I read *The Stress of Life*, by Hans Selye, who defined stress as the nonspecific response of the body to any demand made upon it. I started to evaluate my life and see how much stress I was really experiencing. I work a full time job and have a business, as well as my two kids and a dog. My life is full, but full of mostly good things. Overall my relationships and work life were good and I would not consider myself to have a particularly stressful life.

What I did not take into consideration is that stress can be a physiological response as well, and after reading the work of biologist Ray Peat, I learned eating zero carbohydrates can in fact, be stressful on the body. In his research, Peat writes about the body needing a certain amount of glucose to keep the body from using its lean tissue as fuel. In ketogenic work, this process - called gluconeogenesis - is considered a prized function that helps us to keep our ketones high and in a state of fat burning.

This was the only thing that made sense to me. For two and a half years, I had consumed almost zero carbohydrates. My body was making glucose out of my own tissues and running along pretty well, there was no sign of distress at first. This was a rabbit hole I was going down to understand what was causing my body to shift into this stressed state. I'd had insomnia many times, and at times felt anxious. Both of these worsened with fasting. I was putting my body under a lot of stress by depriving it of calories and glucose, but I didn't associate them with my diet. Sometimes we can't see the trees when we are in the forest.

I learned from Dr. Peat that not having glucose puts stress on the body, and can diminish thyroid functions. Since most of the thyroid hormone made is T4, the body mostly uses T3 which is converted by the liver with the help of glucose. When glucose is lacking, the conversion does not happen as well and T3 levels can quickly drop. Symptoms of low T3 include fatigue, feeling cold, weight gain, dry brittle hair and nails, low libido and even some anxiety. Bingo! The picture was becoming clearer.

In Broda Barnes's book *Hypothyroidism, the Unsuspecting Illness*, I learned about hypothyroidism and how to check my thyroid, with some degree of accuracy though the body temperature and pulse rate. Dr. Barnes had used a standard temperature of 97.8 upon waking, and 98.6 after meals as the minimum temperatures humans should maintain. He also used the pulse rate standard range of 75-95 for those with no thyroid problems, anything lower often correlated with hypothyroidism.

I started monitoring my daily temperature and pulse. The first day I took my temperature: it was 96 degrees, my pulse was 70. I thought this would be a good place to start monitoring for my next experiment in self-study. I was about to add carbohydrates back into my diet in hopes of feeling my energy levels return and I decided to use my self check of temperature and pulse as my measurement. The variable would be glucose, in the form of fruit. I had intense cravings for fruit, my body was begging for it, and I was excited to give in to it. I was a little nervous about how my body would respond to the newly introduced food, but I was excited to give it a try. I told myself that my gut health was most important, and that if I had any symptoms back to carnivore I would go. As a side note, a carnivore diet can easily be done with some carbs in the form of milk and honey although I think fruits have been a critical piece to balancing hormones. I have not liked milk since drinking it warm on the farm, but I was willing to try it. In California, raw milk is hard to find, so I focused on yogurt, fruit and honey as my first additions.

After slowly incorporating berries and papaya, I was feeling more energized and had the best sleep in years. My stomach felt great, I was happy, energized and rested. I did gain around 5 lbs with the sudden influx of glucose, but I knew it was mainly water and would happily trade it for better sleep.

After a few short weeks I introduced more foods in the form of vegetables. I started with mushrooms, which I cooked in butter. Ray Peat had recommended it in many of his interviews as a way to disinfect the bowels along with raw carrots. He said that not only do they help to clear toxins from the bowels but they also remove used estrogens and prevent them from being reabsorbed in the body. Since my labs showed excess estrogen, I knew this would be a good add. I cooked them well in coconut oil and they became a staple alongside my grass fed beef and lamb. The raw carrot I consumed daily, sometimes with coconut oil and vinegar, but most days just rinsed and eaten as a snack while I worked. Carrots contain an indigestible fiber and as they pass through the digestive tract they collect and carry out estrogen that could otherwise be reabsorbed into the colon.

Since my previous labs showed excess estrogen, extremely high cortisol and no testosterone, I was most interested in getting these balanced. Other than poor sleep and anxiety, I could not tell any marked symptoms of having hormones imbalanced but I wanted to improve my numbers to see what the potential was. My foods focused on estrogen antagonists, clearing colon of estrogens and reducing cortisol. I had the first part mostly covered by carrots and mushrooms, but I later learned that fresh squeezed orange juice was one of the best foods to get that estrogen out of the body while also helping the thyroid function better. It turns out, orange juice contains a few compounds that help block estrogen such as apigenin and naringenin. These help to block and remove estrogens from the body so that they do not contribute to health problems such as inflammation, weight gain, cancer and PMS symptoms.

Estrogens do play a role in gut health as well. When there is excess estrogen, not only is it inflammatory, but it also reduces the conversion of T4 into the more usable T3. When thyroid function slows, more estrogen can accumulate, creating a more inflammatory cycle.

An article in *Maturitas*, an international *Journal of Midlife Health And Beyond* stated that "The alteration in circulating estrogens may contribute to the development of conditions discussed herein: obesity, metabolic syndrome, cancer, endometrial hyperplasia, endometriosis, polycystic ovary syndrome, fertility, cardiovascular disease (CVD) and cognitive function."[2829]

Estrogens influence immune and inflammatory processes, as revealed by increased inflammatory responses to infection and sepsis and higher rate of autoimmune diseases in women when compared to men as well as by the variation of chronic inflammatory disease activity with the menstrual cycle, pregnancy, and menopause.

To get my testosterone up I would need to get my cortisol down. Stress from my work, having a busy life and air pollution here in California were things I over which had very little control. I could work on other things though, like sleep and nutrition. My sleep was terrible before adding fruits, so that was well on its way to being solved. Nutrition was more about getting the glucose and enough calories my body needed to keep from catabolizing itself.

It turns out low glucose results in gluconeogenesis and low blood sugar in general raises cortisol. For many years I had been undereating and over exercising, it just became a normal way of life for me. Now, though, the combination was catching up. I was feeling it in the form of hormone imbalance, fatigue and having a really hard time putting on muscle despite working out several days per week.

After nine short months of eating fruit, eating more often and more in general, things started to shift. My blood work revealed that my testosterone had doubled and my cortisol was coming down to reasonable levels. I still had excess estrogen, which I now believe MOST people do, but I was working on it. I also learned that my free T3 hormone was quite low. Free T3 is the thyroid hormone mainly used by your body. The thyroid makes mostly T4, which is then converted to T3 or reverse T3 in the liver and in the gut.

Without enough free T3 we may experience symptoms such as fatigue, depression, feeling cold, poor sleep, weight gain and dry skin and hair. I was experiencing many of these, and I learned that the healthy range for Free T3 was 2-9 ng/ml. Mine was 2.1. Still very low. I was either not converting to T3 or I was creating too much reverse T3, which comes from stress. People under a lot of stress tend to convert more to RT3. I had put myself under a great deal of stress over the previous couple of years with zero carbohydrates, too low calories, and long periods without eating. I had solved my major digestive disease, but lost some thyroid function in the process.

Studying Dr. Ray Peat has been very eye opening. Much like the carnivore experience, I learned that many things we are *taught* to be unhealthy are actually some of the healthiest things for us. We have been told for years that saturated fats are dangerous. Then we learned this was not at all the case, and in fact it was the *unsaturated* fats that do the harm.

We were told that salt was unhealthy and we should not use it on our foods, but it turns out salt is actually necessary for proper hormone balance, especially during stress. The next big lie to unravel was the one about sugar. All my life I had believed sugar was the worst thing for my health. I avoided it like a poison for the better part of 20 years. What I learned from Dr. Ray Peat was that it actually supports the thyroid, which is a master gland of the body. When thyroid function fails, many other areas of health go awry.

Since I live a somewhat stressful life as do most people, managing it to protect my thyroid will likely be an ongoing piece of the health puzzle. If thyroid function is low, estrogen dominance in any form can result. If we are estrogen dominant we have uncomfortable symptoms but also run a much higher risk of chronic diseases including cancer. We can gain weight, have poor sleep, and even suffer mental illness as a result of low thyroid function. After all the work I have done to heal my gut, I certainly will not fall into another chronic illness that is within my control. If eating sugar means a healthy thyroid, so be it. Luckily, it can be a very healthy form of sugar that supports us most. Fruit has been my go-to and is also the best source of carbohydrates recommended by Dr. Peat. Most fruits are easy to digest and contain a host of helpful minerals and fructose to help the thyroid by keeping the stress hormones low.

Again, the diet dogma had haunted me and brainwashed me to believe that sugar was bad, even natural fruits. I will admit I had adopted this belief wholeheartedly, just as I had with veganism, (fat is bad etc). I suppose when we know better we can do better, but incorporating more glucose in the form of fruits and even honey has made a world of difference for my health. I was finally feeling healthy and balanced in ALL areas of life.

As I write this book I am now four years past my experience with ulcerative colitis. I would call myself healed, however others might call this remission. Since my symptoms ceased, just 4 months into the carnivore diet, I have still not had any symptoms whatsoever.

I continue to improve on my health by eating an animal based diet high in calcium, protein and fresh fruits, along with wild caught seafood, grass fed meats and pasture raised chicken and eggs. I am acutely aware of additives in foods and steer clear of them as I now believe they are a major contributor of gut damage. I currently have no health complaints, however I continue to improve on my supportive diet and mitigation of stress.

I don't believe anyone is immune to the perils of gut damage since most people are exposed to some degree of irritating foods, toxins and stress. It may only be a matter of time for many people before a chronic illness arises. What I see most often in people who reach out to me for help, is that regardless of their health condition, they usually have the same underlying gut issues whether they know it or not. In Part 2, I will explain exactly how many health conditions are actually gut problems in disguise, and how you can regain your health by starting there. The cause of many illnesses starts with gut health, but it is also the cure.

---

[16]https://www.ncbi.nlm.nih.gov/pmc/articles/PMC7600777/
[17] http://raypeat.com/articles/articles/fats-functions-malfunctions.shtml
[18] https://usrtk.org/pesticides/glyphosate-use-in-food-crops/
[19]https://www.ncbi.nlm.nih.gov/pmc/articles/PMC3945755/
[20] https://www.aamc.org/media/25711/download
[21]https://pdfs.semanticscholar.org/0a01/8eef2c4d4516b21ee822
44508eb75edaa7af.pdf
[22] https://www.gastrojournal.org/article/S0016-5085(18)30018-

0/fulltext
[23] https://www.hindawi.com/journals/jbe/2015/357627/
[24] https://pubmed.ncbi.nlm.nih.gov/26234947/
[25] https://now.tufts.edu/news-releases/report-card-diet-trends-low-quality-carbs-account-42-percent-day-s-calories
[26] http://raypeat.com/articles/articles/vegetables.shtml
[27]https://www.dropbox.com/s/jfmhar9xl9zuj7x/Screen%20Shot%202021-07-24%20at%202.26.55%20PM.png?dl=0
[28] https://www.maturitas.org/article/S0378-5122(17)30650-3/fulltext
[29] Baker JM, Al-Nakkash L, Herbst-Kralovetz MM. *Estrogen-gut microbiome axis: Physiological and clinical implications.* *Maturitas.* 2017 Sep;103:45-53. doi: 10.1016/j.maturitas.2017.06.025. Epub 2017 Jun 23. PMID: 28778332.

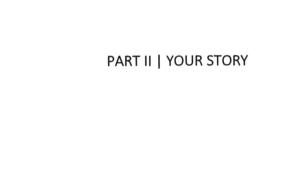

PART II | YOUR STORY

ONE: YOUR HEALTH DEPENDS ON THE GUT

Now that you have heard my story, I want to share with you some of the research that links many chronic diseases to the health of your gut. You are about to see how the gut does so much more than digest and process food. It is one of the most important factors in the health outcomes of so many conditions.

In my coaching practice, I see men and women with many different health concerns. They often wish to lose weight, clear their acne, balance their hormones or simply to feel better. I know that these are common requests among people, and that there is a reason why so many people struggle in these areas.

One example is a young woman who hired me to help improve her adult acne, which she had for many years. When we had our first meeting, she explained the hundreds of different skin care products she had tried over the years, even antibiotics, in an effort to clear her skin. She described the various supplements and pills she took, and that although some helped slightly, she could never really resolve the problem. When I asked her if she has even worked on gut health, her only answer was that she took probiotics. We worked on figuring out what might be irritating her gut, and uncovered more symptoms that had simply become her "normal" state. We removed the irritants, strengthened her gut and addressed some stress she was having. Her skin was clear within two months of working with me. I never once suggested any kind of cream, lotion or potion - just working on the gut.

In another case, I worked with a young woman who was having severe depression and digestive problems. She had been taking SSRI and was unhappy with the bothersome side effects, and was indeed still depressed. Through our work together, we were able to identify a very specific item in her very strict diet (black pepper) that was inflaming her gut, and when she removed it from her diet, the depression lifted. I have witnessed a similar thing happen with several others.

I also worked with the daughter of a friend, who since infancy, had been diagnosed with oppositional behavior and struggled with anxiety, depression and ADD. She was born with severe gut damage, severe respiratory conditions, eczema and was labeled "failure to thrive" at 6 months old due to her inability to gain weight. She would have frequent meltdowns, hours long screaming fits almost daily. The mother was in distress from lack of sleep and the emotional toll it was taking on her. By the time the baby was 2, she was underweight and had rotting teeth due to severe acid reflux. She had her first endoscopy at 7 months. She had been to several doctors and was given a variety of antacids and later proton pump inhibitors, but still could not gain weight and would barely eat. I strongly felt she was having a food intolerance, and she was tested for food allergies and the like, which came out "off the charts" positive for Celiac. At age 5 she started a gluten free diet.

We worked on eliminating foods that could cause irritation, and soon she began to calm down, sleep and finally gain weight. Once the irritants were fully removed, she improved within two weeks, and within a month the symptoms were entirely reversed. Her mom and I are best friends today.

When I ask people if they think they have problems with their gut, they say "no" unless they have a very obvious digestive disorder such as ulcerative colitis. However, those same people struggle with anxiety, depression, asthma, insomnia, skin troubles, immune dysfunction, and other autoimmune disorders that they simply do not associate with the gut. This is understandable, because in Western medicine and culture, we have a very finite connection between a symptom and an illness. For example, a headache is only a pain in the head, nothing more, and only needs to be solved with ibuprofen. This is how many ailments are treated, without looking further into addressing the cause of the headache. The same can be true for digestive health. If you have ulcerative colitis, it will be recommended that you use anti-inflammatory agents to reduce the inflammation in the colon, or remove the colon entirely, rather than understanding what could be driving the inflammation and working on that.

As I have mentioned previously, our food supply is filled with toxins from farming and poor water quality, genetic engineering of food and soil that lacks nutrients. Foods that are considered healthy are made of soy, beans, grains and other plants that contain many irritants. In addition, we have more processed foods in the world than ever in history, and many are even considered "health foods" such as protein bars, salad dressings and dairy alternatives.

Eating has become a war zone for someone who WANTS to choose healthy, and an absolute tragedy for those that believe food is food.

Unfortunately, our medical system does not often address the gut unless specific gut-related symptoms are present - and even in that case they are usually treated with drugs (to mitigate symptoms) or surgery to remove the offending organ such as the gallbladder, appendix or even the colon.

The health of our gut is impacted by our food, lifestyle, toxins, stress, and trauma in our lives, and no drug or surgery can fix that.

How Does Our Gut Become Damaged?

There are many things that can cause gut permeability, essentially it is a result of a stressor. Stress can be caused by a toxin, a thought, an illness. It can be chemical, physical, or emotional. Some of the stress triggers for gut damage can include a traumatic event, extreme dieting and exercise, excessive vegetable intake, or exposure to toxins.

Some of the triggers for gut damage can include a traumatic event, extreme dieting, excessive vegetable intake or exposure to toxins. In a 2014 paper published in *Autoimmune Diseases*, the author acknowledges that there are a "vast number" of environmental toxins that can trigger autoimmune disease including chemicals, bacteria, viruses and mold. He also points out that since World War II the amount of autoimmune diseases has increased to pandemic levels and coincides with the simultaneous increase of agricultural chemicals as well.[30]

One area of concern are Persistent Organic Pollutants (also known as POPs) that became common practice after

World War II. These are found mostly in contaminated foods and water. POPs are intentionally made chemicals for use in agriculture to control pests and diseases in crops and also in machinery used in processing such as lubricants. The most notable POPs include polychlorinated biphenyls (PCBs), DDT and also include dioxins which are a byproduct of the combustion of waste. Thougt DDT has long since been discontinued in the United States it is still used in other countries where it can and does make its way to the US by way of air and dust where it continues to pollute our land, air and water. Animals grazing on contaminated farmland can also store these chemicals in their fat cells making their way to humans through the food supply. This form of biomagnification results in those that are at the top of the food chain (humans) ingest the highest concentrations of chemicals.

These concerns were addressed in 2001 with the signing of the Stockholm Convention, the global collaboration of countries to commit to the ban of use of POP's in order to trade agricultural goods to protect humans and wildlife. Unfortunately not all countries took part, and some of these chemicals are still used today. To make matters worse, the POP's can persist in the environment, once released, for hundreds of years.

Interestingly, one of the areas of the US hardest hit were the Great Lakes. All five of the lakes were found to be highly contaminated with a variety of POPs, heavy metals, and other agricultural and industrial pollutants. In 1972, The US and Canada signed the Great Lakes Water Quality Agreement to control pollution, banning the release of these chemicals into the lakes. They have continued to monitor their contamination levels since 1990, but unfortunately they still today contain high levels of POPs and heavy metals. At the center of the Great Lakes is Michigan, the state where I grew up, swimming, boating and fishing every summer.[31]

Other possible causes of gut damage and dysbiosis are antibiotics. In a 2020 paper published in *The Critical Reviews in Food Science Nutrition*, it is very clearly spelled out that antibiotics used both in humans and animals can inevitably cause gut dysbiosis and barrier disruption. If we understand that the mucosal lining is a critical piece of protection to the gut wall, then we can also understand that damaging it will have serious implications to our gut. The article states "The intestinal barrier, which comprises secretory, physical, and immunological barriers, is also a target of antibiotics. Antibiotic induced changes in the gut microbiota composition could induce weakening of the gut barrier through changes in mucin, cytokine, and antimicrobial peptide production by intestinal epithelial cells." It goes on to say that dietary measures such as using prebiotics, probiotics and butyrate can mitigate some of the effects of antibiotics on the gut lining.[3233]

The overuse of antibiotics is well known, and had been a topic of concern since I was in graduate school in 2003. We were given the ungrateful job of going door to door at local medical centers, handing out information leaflets to physicians on the dangers of overusing antibiotics. They never took us seriously (silly grad students), and promptly threw the leaflets in the trash in most cases. The World Health Organization now calls it "one of the biggest threats to global health, food security, and development today."[34]

Antibiotics aren't the only drug that can harm the gut. Proton pump inhibitors, or PPIs, used to reduce acid reflux can also alter the gut microbiome and reduce natural digestive acids, causing indigestion and promoting endotoxins. A human study published in the *British Medical Journal* found that those in the study who took PPIs were consistently associated with changes towards a less healthy gut microbiome as compared to the control subjects.[35]

A 2018 study published in the journal *Nature* stated that one quarter of all medications have a negative impact on gut health, not just antibiotics. These medications affect both good bacteria and pathogens alike. The study found that drugs including antivirals, antipsychotics, acid-reducing medications, chemotherapy drugs, and blood-pressure medications all inhibited the growth of healthy bacteria.[36]

Even the most common over-the-counter drug, such as ibuprofen, has implications on gut health. A 2015 study on the effects of medications on the human gut microbiome found changes in microbiome when participants used NSAIDs, antibiotics and antidepressants.[37]

Other commonly used drugs that were shown to affect gut health include metformin, laxatives, and tetracyclines.[38]

Even birth control pills have been implicated in gut lining damage due to the estrogenic effect causing inflammatory bowel disease. Using birth control can increase your risk of developing Crohn's disease and ulcerative colitis.[39]

Not everyone will have the same telltale signs of gut damage. In fact, some people notice no digestive issues whatsoever, but they have other health problems or chronic diseases that are difficult to treat. In the next chapters, we'll cover these.

---

[30]https://www.ncbi.nlm.nih.gov/pmc/articles/PMC4036413/

[31] https://www.epa.gov/international-cooperation/persistent-organic-pollutants-global-issue-global-response#table

[32] https://pubmed.ncbi.nlm.nih.gov/33198506/

[33] Duan H, Yu L, Tian F, Zhai Q, Fan L, Chen W. *Antibiotic-induced gut dysbiosis and barrier disruption and the potential protective strategies. Crit Rev Food Sci Nutr. 2020 Nov 16*:1-26. doi: 10.1080/10408398.2020.1843396. Epub ahead of print. PMID: 33198506

[34] https://www.who.int/news-room/fact-sheets/detail/antibiotic-resistance

[35] https://gut.bmj.com/content/65/5/740

[36]https://www.theguardian.com/science/2018/mar/19/wide-range-of-drugs-affect-gut-microbes-not-just-antibiotics

[37]https://www.ncbi.nlm.nih.gov/pmc/articles/PMC4754147/

[38]https://www.ncbi.nlm.nih.gov/pmc/articles/PMC6969170/

[39]https://www.ncbi.nlm.nih.gov/pmc/articles/PMC4752384/

TWO: AUTOIMMUNE DISEASE

Autoimmune disease occurs when the body's immune system attacks its own healthy organs and tissues instead of infectious agents. They are extremely common in recent years, and affect nearly 24 million Americans.[40]

Women are affected more than men when it comes to autoimmune disease in fact they are among the leading causes of death among young and middle-aged women in the United States, and are among the top 10 causes of death among females.[41] I find this very interesting, because women are notoriously MORE engaged than men in their health care. They typically engage in healthier habits, participate in preventative screenings, and exercise more. Women live longer than men, and they also verbalize many illnesses more than men - which may result in the treatment and health conditions being addressed more often and earlier than in men.[42] This could be attributed to the closer connection to health care, but I have often wondered if there is a connection between the higher vegetable consumption in women, and the increased rate of autoimmune disease. Could our agricultural practices contribute to chemical overload via vegetable consumption? Some researchers have suggested it has to do with the placenta a woman carries, the fact that women have two X chromosomes, and other genetic hypotheses.[43]

There are more than 80 different types of autoimmune disease. Common autoimmune diseases include celiac disease, psoriasis, Inflammatory Bowel Disease, Hashimoto's Thyroiditis, Lupus, Type 1 Diabetes, Rheumatoid Arthritis, Graves Disease and Crohn's Disease to name a few. Autoimmune diseases are so varied that people are often diagnosed with an autoimmune disease when no other diagnosis can be found to explain their condition. Physicians use this autoinflammatory condition to describe a recurring immune response with no known origin - which essentially means they have no idea what the cause is. What we do know is that in all of these cases, the immune system is responding to a threat.[44]

Most medical literature regarding autoimmune disease will state that there is no known cause of autoimmune disease, however "leaky gut" is present in many different autoimmune conditions. Autoimmune diseases are still considered to have an unknown cause or origin, however in the naturopathic community it is generally accepted that most are related to a leaky gut. The leaky gut theory, also known as gut permeability, is a condition where the tight junctions of the lining of the gut become inflamed, and eventually separate creating microscopic openings in the lining of the gut. This is dangerous because that lining is supposed to separate the contents of your digestive system from the bloodstream. When particles can pass from these microscopic openings into the bloodstream, the body sees it as an invasive material and creates an inflammatory response to protect the body. This inflammation can spread to many other organs and tissues of the body. For all autoimmune diseases, the state of that organ is usually inflammation and this may be its source.

The mainstream medical model is beginning to recognize the relationship between gut health and autoimmune disease. According to a 2017 paper in In Frontiers in Immunology, "individuals with a genetic predisposition, a leaky gut may allow environmental factors to enter the body and trigger the initiation and development of autoimmune disease." The article points to a disruption in microbiome as the trigger to losing protection of the intestinal lining, which puts one at risk of a leaky gut. The article also points out pathogenic bacteria that can facilitate a leaky gut and induce autoimmune symptoms.[45]

Genetic predisposition, environmental factors and gut dysbiosis play major roles in the development of autoimmune diseases. These are broad categories that can include many things. Toxins, heavy metals, viruses and medications are all implicated as possible triggers of autoimmune disease. New research on several autoimmune diseases point to imbalances within the gut microbiome or a damaged gut as a major contributor to the onset of disease.

Rheumatoid Arthritis

A 2013 study conducted at NYU School of Medicine found that 75% of individuals with new-onset RA had a specific type of bacteria in their microbiome called Prevotella copri that has an influence on inflammation. Although the researchers can't say the bacteria causes RA, it may very well be part of the puzzle.[46]

*

Hashimoto's Thyroiditis

Hashimoto's thyroiditis is the most frequent autoimmune disease worldwide. In the June 2020 edition of the journal Nutrients reported that dysbiosis was found not only in Hashimoto's Thyroiditis patients, but also in patients with thyroid cancer. Many of the nutrients needed for a healthy thyroid such as selenium, zinc, copper and iodine are also deficient in those with a compromised gut microbiota.[47]

Another literature review in 2018 stated that there is evidence the genesis and progression of autoimmune thyroid disorders may be significantly affected from a changing intestinal microbial composition, or even from overt dysbiosis.[48]

Graves' Disease

Graves' disease is another thyroid disorder where the thyroid becomes overactive. Patients of Graves' disease often have a rapid heart beat, overactive digestion, heat sensitivity, nervousness or irritability, trouble sleeping, fatigue, and weight loss. People who have other autoimmune diseases are more susceptible to Graves' disease. It affects about 1 in 200 people and is thought to be genetic, or caused by a virus.[49]

A 2021 study showed that patients with Graves' disease fecal samples had significantly lower *firmicutes* and significantly higher *bacteroidetes*, and had less microbiome diversity than did healthy subjects.[50]

In those with Graves' disease, researchers consistently found elevated levels of a bacteria called *Actinomyces_odontolyticus,* which is also involved with other diseases including periodontal disease and colorectal cancer.[51]

A 2020 review stated that Graves' disease is often accompanied by celiac disease and can be explained by a damaged intestinal barrier.[52]

Celiac Disease

Celiac disease is an autoimmune disease where those with a genetic predisposition have reactions to any foods with gluten such as wheat, rye or oats. Johns Hopkins medical center calls celiac disease a genetic disorder that results in the immune system attacking the villi, or lining of the gut, and preventing the absorption of certain nutrients. Although it is considered genetic, it may be triggered by stress on the body such as in injury, surgery, infection, pregnancy or other major stress. People with celiac disease often have constipation or diarrhea, foul-smelling stools, gas, bloating, weight loss and anemia among other things.[53]

In a 2019 study published in the *Human Microbiome Journal*, the authors stated that their research suggests that changes in the blood microbiome may contribute to the pathogenesis of celiac disease.[54]

Type 1 Diabetes

Type 1 diabetes is an autoimmune disease in which little to no insulin is produced in the pancreas. People with Type 1 Diabetes have very high blood sugar levels along with increased thirst and urination, fatigue, weight loss and slow healing from wounds. Like other autoimmune diseases, the cause is unknown but may have environmental factors. Recent research is uncovering a link between the microbiome and triggering of these environmental factors.[55]

Type 2 diabetes may also be related to microbiome. The metabolites from the gut microbes contribute to the gut barrier and a compromised barrier leads to leakage of inflammatory mediators into systemic circulation and hence increases insulin resistance.[56]

A 2020 study done on individuals of Northern China found an increase in *firmicutes* abundance and a relatively lower abundance of *bacteroidetes* were found in diabetic subjects.[57]

Vitiligo and Alopecia

Vitiligo is characterized by the loss of pigment in the skin causing white patches to appear on the body and is among the most common autoimmune diseases. It can show up on certain areas of the body such as only the face, or only the legs or even on only one side of the body. The cause is unknown as with other autoimmune diseases but stress of some kind, especially to the skin (such as a burn), is thought to be a major trigger. A study done with mice found that, when given an antibiotic they were ⅓ depigmented in 30 weeks as opposed to a control group who received no treatment. This points to a connection between gut microbiome and vitiligo, but does not give clear results as to how to prevent or treat it in humans.[58]

Alopecia is the autoimmune disease that causes hair loss on the head, or over the entire body. It can fall out in patches, all at once, or gradually over time. Certain conditions such as cold temperatures, can worsen hair loss. An interesting study done with mice and probiotics showed that mice given *Lactobacillus murinus*, the mice lost nearly all of their hair. When they were given the same bacteria with biotin, they had no hair loss demonstrating that diet, along with bacteria in the gut, may prevent hair loss.[59]

A human alopecia study, done at University of California Irvine in 2020, tested a group of individuals with alopecia by testing their scalp and fecal microbiome and comparing them to healthy individuals. Researchers found that it varies greatly from healthy individuals with no hair loss.[60]

These are just a few examples of common autoimmune diseases that have been studied for their relationship to the microbiome and gut health. Although we don't have all the answers yet, they all seem to point to some relationship with the gut.

Traditional treatment for autoimmune disease depends on the type a person has, but in most cases will be addressed with drugs that suppress the immune system. For example, typical treatments for inflammatory bowel diseases are anti-inflammatory medications, antibiotics and biologics such as Remicade that neutralizes proteins called tumor necrosis factor. Nutritional support is only focused on supporting one's body weight as many people with inflammatory bowel disease get very thin. Sometime's vitamin and mineral supplementation or IV will be given as many patients with bowel disease are unable to absorb nutrients properly.

As more research becomes available, demonstrating the different types of gut bacteria and their effect on autoimmunity, we may see gut health becoming a more targeted approach in the near future. For now, all we can do is support the gut in hopes for improvement. People deserve better than an onslaught of drugs that have many side effects. More time and attention needs to be paid to what we now know has a major impact on autoimmune disease, and may even hold the cure for many people.

[40] https://www.hopkinsmedicine.org/health/wellness-and-prevention/autoimmune-disease-why-is-my-immune-system-attacking-itself

[41] https://pubmed.ncbi.nlm.nih.gov/12848952/

[42] https://pubmed.ncbi.nlm.nih.gov/3213237/

[43] https://www.cell.com/trends/genetics/fulltext/S0168-9525(19)30079-4

[44] https://www.niaid.nih.gov/diseases-conditions/autoimmune-diseases

[45] https://www.ncbi.nlm.nih.gov/pmc/articles/PMC5440529/

[46] https://www.nih.gov/news-events/nih-research-matters/gut-microbes-linked-rheumatoid-arthritis

[47]https://www.ncbi.nlm.nih.gov/pmc/articles/PMC7353203/

[48] Virili C, Fallahi P, Antonelli A, Benvenga S, Centanni M. *Gut microbiota and Hashimoto's thyroiditis. Rev Endocr Metab Disord. 2018 Dec*;19(4):293-300. doi: 10.1007/s11154-018-9467-y. PMID: 30294759

[49] https://www.niddk.nih.gov/health-information/endocrine-diseases/graves-disease

[50]https://www.ncbi.nlm.nih.gov/pmc/articles/PMC8110022/

[51]https://www.frontiersin.org/articles/10.3389/fcimb.2021.663131/full

[52] https://pubmed.ncbi.nlm.nih.gov/32545596/

[53] https://www.hopkinsmedicine.org/health/conditions-and-diseases/celiac-disease

[54]https://www.sciencedirect.com/science/article/pii/S2452231718300368

[55] https://www.ncbi.nlm.nih.gov/pmc/articles/PMC6220847/

[56] https://pubmed.ncbi.nlm.nih.gov/25901889/

[57] https://www.nature.com/articles/s41598-020-62224-3

[58] https://pubmed.ncbi.nlm.nih.gov/31472106/

[59] https://jofskin.org/index.php/skin/article/view/719

[60] https://jofskin.org/index.php/skin/article/view/719

THREE: MENTAL HEALTH

The microbiome has been linked to a wide range of mental health conditions including autism, anxiety, depression, insomnia, Alzheimers and even one's personality. In recent years, the number of studies published on gut microbiome with regards to mental health has skyrocketed. There is a microbiota that is specific to the nerves and the brain that has been coined as the "psychobiota" by scientists John Cryan and Ted Dinan. These microbes influence chemicals in the brain and inflammation, prompting cells in the gut lining to stimulate the vagus nerve and activate endocrine cells in the gut that secrete the hormones that are released in the body.[61]

This is, in my opinion, one of the most exciting and interesting areas within the study of gut health - mainly because millions of people suffer with mental illness, and most of them are only given the option of drugs to help them cope. According to the National Alliance on Mental Illness, 20.6% of U.S. adults, or 1 in 5, experienced mental illness in 2019. That is over 50 million people in the United States alone.[62]

What is more tragic - is the average person with a mental illness waits years before seeking treatment and 70% of individuals around the world get no treatment at all for their mental illness. This may be due mostly because of the stigma associated with mental illness but also for fear of being a target of discrimination. Many people with mental health issues do not know that they can be treated - if they do, they may think there are few options in the way of treatment or few places to get care.[63]

Mental illness includes health conditions involving changes in emotion, thinking or behavior and are associated with distress and/or problems functioning in social, work or family activities. Mental illness can adversely affect a person's life, and in major ways.[64]

Mental illness is often treated with cognitive behavioral therapy and medication. It is sometimes also treated with complementary and alternative medicine, but rarely is it approached as a gut health problem. That may be changing. In 2019, the *Canadian Journal of Psychiatry* published a paper discussing the gut microbiome as a potential therapeutic target for mental illness. In fact, I was happily surprised to read that patients with psychiatric disorders have been shown to have significant differences in the composition of their gut microbiome. The author also wrote that enhancing beneficial bacteria in the gut has the potential to improve mood and to reduce anxiety.[65]

Psychiatric conditions that may respond to dietary changes and probiotics include depression, bipolar disorder, schizophrenia, and autism spectrum disorder. All show differences in their gut microbiome as compared to those who do not have these mental health conditions, which may indicate the potential for microbiome targeted therapy as a possible treatment. A study as recent as May 2020 showed that probiotics, live organisms that when administered in adequate amounts, offer health benefits to the host, were effective for depression and improving mood through the gut-brain axis.[66]

This brings hope to disorders of the gut-brain axis. If the microbiome is affected enough by probiotics to improve depression, maybe there is a chance other things that affect the microbiome can also improve other psychiatric conditions. This area of research is a very hot topic and newspapers are coming out all of the time. We are onto something here, and my experience with changes in mood (without taking probiotics) seem to point to just that. Still, we are waiting for more definitive answers to come through research to help guide providers in helping their patients with mood disorders and other mental health challenges.

All of this is zeroing in on the connection between the gastrointestinal tract and the central nervous system, also referred to as the gut-brain axis. This gut-brain axis is how the brain communicates with the gut, and how the gut communicates with the brain. It includes the gut microbiome, the vagus nerve, the enteric nervous system, the hypothalamic-pituitary-adrenal (HPA) axis as well as both the sympathetic and parasympathetic nervous system.[67]

All of this may sound overwhelming, but the message is simple: the gut is not just for digestion, but it interacts with your brain and all of your nervous system. This, in a nutshell, is the reason gut health so profoundly affects other areas of health.

---

[61] https://nnia.nestlenutrition-

institute.org/news/article/2021/07/09/could-gut-microbiome-hold-key-mental-health

[62] https://www.nami.org/mhstats

[63] https://www.ncbi.nlm.nih.gov/pmc/articles/PMC3698814/

[64] https://www.psychiatry.org/patients-families/what-is-mental-illness

[65] https://pubmed.ncbi.nlm.nih.gov/31530002/

[66] https://www.ncbi.nlm.nih.gov/pmc/articles/PMC7398953/

[67] https://en.wikipedia.org/wiki/Gut%E2%80%93brain_axis

FOUR: SKIN DISORDERS

The skin is the largest organ of the body. Changes in the skin can provide clues as to what is happening inside the body. Skin provides a protective barrier to pathogens, regulates our temperature and provinces us with tactile sensations. The deepest layers of the skin store water, fats and metabolic products. Skin also helps with hormone production. As the deeper layers make new skin cells that are pushed to the surface every 4 weeks, the top layer of the skin - called the epidermis - is constantly renewing itself.[68]

The skin itself has its own microbiome. The microbiome naturally contains bacteria, fungi and viruses that play a role in protecting our skin and our health. This is the first layer of our immune system we have to protect us. In 1930, John H. Stokes and Donald M. Pillsbury proposed the theory that there is a gut-brain-skin axis suggesting that emotional upset can alter the gut which in turn alters the skin. Since then, more recently as microbiome research has boomed, these theories have been validated with the gut-brain axis and the recognition that the skin is directly affected by the gut microbiome. Another theory is that having a leaky gut allows for inflammatory agents to pass from the gut to the bloodstream causing systemic inflammation.[69]

Acne is another one of those chronic health issues with no known cause. The health of the gut microbiome affects the health of the skin microbiome. Who knew! In researching acne for this book, I found the term "gut-skin axis" for the first time. It refers to the bidirectional connection between the gut and the skin. When the gut converts fiber to short chain fatty acids, it feeds the good bacteria in the gut, helping to create a positive balance in the microbiome in both the gut and the skin.[70]

It turns out that the skin is highly sensitive to the changes of the gut microbiome. Depending on the balance of microbes, one might have either normal skin or any number of skin disorders, including acne. Most people address acne with topical preparations to dry it out, but the main target should be the gut. In addition, we must be careful not to disrupt the skin microbiome itself, which chemicals in products used for acne or antibacterial products could do.

A 2019 review in the *Journal of Clinical Medicine* indicated that the gut-brain axis also connects to the skin. It stated that emotions and stress that impact the gut can alter the skin, by disrupting the microbiome.[71]

Rosacea is a persistent flushing or reddening of the skin, usually in the face. It can also cause a burning sensation and swelling in the skin as well as a thickening of the skin over time. Rosacea is considered to be an overactive immune response to certain foods like alcohol, capsaicin (pepper) foods, hot temperature foods, or irritation from the sun. Knowing that it is based on an immune response, we know that the immune system is dependent on the gut, so as with most autoimmune conditions we can start there.

Epidemiological studies show that people with rosacea have higher rates of gastrointestinal disease according to a

2018 paper published in *Dermatology Practical and Conceptual*. Cases where patients were treated for SIBO found improvement in rosacea, indicating a direct link from gut health to the disease.[72]

Psoriasis is a chronic disease characterized by itchy scaly patches of skin across various parts of the body but with a tendency to afflict the scalp, knees, elbows and trunk. There are several forms of psoriasis and it can affect the joints, causing pain and discomfort which interfere with regular life's activities. The cause of psoriasis isn't clear.

A 2020 review, published in *Frontiers in Microbiology*, states "psoriasis, a common chronic inflammatory dermatosis, impacts 1–3% of the world's population. The exact factors that drive psoriasis are not fully understood, but it is considered to be a complicated immune-mediated disease and is affected by both human genetics and environmental factors such as diet, lifestyle and health history."

Since we know how powerfully diet can affect the gut, we can draw some conclusions about the relevance of gut health for psoriasis patients. The authors discuss another study in which Candida species were found to be prevalent on the skin in psoriasis lesions and in the feces of patients with psoriasis.[73]

Pemphigus is a rare disease that causes blistering of the skin and the inside of the mouth, nose, throat, eyes, and genitals due to antibodies against proteins that bind skin cells to one another. When these bonds are disrupted, fluids collect between its layers, forming blisters.[74]

Researchers studied the gut microbiome of patients with pemphigus and found they consistently have gut microbial dysbiosis which might contribute to the immune disorder.[75]

I myself have never had any kind of skin ailments. I have seen many people that do, however, and in those that I have worked with, taking care of the gut gets results. Unfortunately, it doesn't always happen as fast as we would like, but by reducing endotoxins in the gut, feeding it good prebiotics and balancing the hormones, we can accomplish great things for the skin and overall health.

---

[68] https://www.ncbi.nlm.nih.gov/books/NBK279255/
[69] https://www.ncbi.nlm.nih.gov/pmc/articles/PMC6920876/
[70] https://www.ncbi.nlm.nih.gov/pmc/articles/PMC6048199/
[71] https://pubmed.ncbi.nlm.nih.gov/31284694/
[72] https://www.ncbi.nlm.nih.gov/pmc/articles/PMC5718124/
[73] https://www.ncbi.nlm.nih.gov/pmc/articles/PMC7769758/
[74] https://www.niams.nih.gov/health-topics/pemphigus/advanced
[75] https://pubmed.ncbi.nlm.nih.gov/31211854/

FIVE: DIGESTIVE DISORDERS

Since so many diseases are linked to gut damage, it goes without saying that people may experience some type of digestive dysfunction as well. Although this isn't always the case, we do know that illness related to the digestive system is usually related to inflammation and, oftentimes, autoimmunity. Endotoxins, a gram-positive bacteria that initiates an inflammatory response, are also implicated in some of the most common digestive disorders as well. For those whose gut damage or microbiome imbalance shows up as a digestive disease, there are a variety of digestive problems which can unfold.

Some people with gut damage have clearly defined gastrointestinal symptoms and fall under the category of inflammatory bowel disease. Some research has found that IBD patients with Crohn's or ulcerative colitis have, in most cases, a thinner mucosal lining - which is considered to be a protective barrier to the gut wall. How is this lining damaged? And what other factors might be causing this problem?

Inflammatory bowel disease refers to both ulcerative colitis and Crohn's disease, which are chronic autoimmune diseases causing inflammation to the colon and intestines.

Ulcerative colitis is the disease that I had, and it is the inflammation of a portion of - or the entire - colon. Oftentimes, the colon walls have ulcerations which flare up and bleed causing increased bleeding, pain and sometimes diarrhea. As mentioned in Part 1, there is no known cause of the disease, but it is considered to be an autoimmune disease. Some studies suggest that the imbalance in the microbiome causes inflammation, which impairs your epithelial cells in the gut lining.[76]

Food additives are another factor in the development of ulcerative colitis. Carrageenan, a common thickener used in foods, is actually used to INDUCE ulcerative colitis in rats that are to be used in the study of the disease.[77]

Both aluminium and titanium dioxide, given to chemically induced rats with colitis, worsen their condition. Aluminum can be found in food and beauty care products. Titanium dioxide is found in processed foods as a whitener, toothpaste, chewing gum, coffee creamer, chocolates and candies but is "generally regarded as safe" (GRAS) by the FDA.[78]

The diversity of the microbiome has been shown to affect the health of the gut, as ulcerative colitis patients had less diversity in their gut than those with a healthy gut. In our overly hygienic society, humans have lower exposures to microbes that help develop the immune system.

Less diversity in the microbiome may also mean less bacteria that helps feed butyrate. The bacteria that feed butyrate, called *firmicutes*, are lower in people with inflammatory bowel disease than in healthy people. Butyrate helps to protect the mucosal lining of the gut. Butyrate also inhibits inflammation in the gut while strengthening the epithelial cells of the gut and colon, protecting the tight junctions in the colon wall and preventing leakiness of the gut, also known as gut permeability.[7980]

The cause of Crohn's disease is also unknown but even the NIH states that antibiotics, NSIADS like aspirin and high fat diets can be a possible cause. Interestingly, while researching antibiotic use as being a possible cause of ulcerative colitis, there are no scientific papers alluding to that fact; however, I do know at least one person who developed ulcerative colitis within a few weeks of taking a large dose of antibiotics. Even though the scientific evidence may not be there, we can not ignore the anecdotal evidence.[81]

A question that we often have: why don't we all experience this disease if inflammation of the intestines is so common? Shouldn't we all have the same response? Researchers at Emory University say that our immune system should be able to accommodate inflammation to the gut but in some cases, if the immune system is not functioning properly, it isn't able to do its job and further problems arise. According to their paper published in 2012 they say that "Breakdown of the intestinal barrier can occur as a result of intestinal infections or stress. The normal response involves several components of the immune system that help to heal the injury while controlling invading bacteria. When this normal response is defective, and there is a leaky barrier, the risk of developing IBD is increased."[82]

Irritable bowel syndrome is yet another digestive disease that may have an autoimmune origin. The cause of the disease is unknown, but it affects approximately 15 million people worldwide. IBS is characterized by alternating symptoms of dry stools and constipation with water stools, bloating, diarrhea, and oftentimes anxiety. A 2018 paper describes the gut microbiome of those with IBS as having less bacterial diversity than those without IBS.[83]

Another very interesting study done in 2017 showed that when germ-free mice were given a fecal transplant colonized with IBS-D they exhibited symptoms of IBS, such as increased stool transit time, intestinal barrier dysfunction and anxiety-like behaviors.[84]

Small Intestinal Bacterial Overgrowth (SIBO) is a common digestive problem where food items that are difficult to digest end up staying in the gut too long and producing an unhealthy bacteria called endotoxin. One study pointed out that SIBO is often initiated by achlorhydria, or low stomach acids, which may be caused by long term use of proton pump inhibitors - causing bacterial overgrowth in the stomach and duodenum.[85]

Reduced motility can also contribute to SIBO. During periods of fasting, a migrating motor complex (MMC) sweeps residual debris through the gastrointestinal tract. Several studies have demonstrated that abnormalities in the MMC may predispose to the development of SIBO. Fasting may be a good strategy to improve that motility, and to allow the migrating motor complex to do its work in keeping the intestines free of debris.[86]

Gastroesophageal Reflux Disease (GERD) is also known as heartburn where stomach acids make their way to the esophagus and over time erode its lining. GERD is often treated with proton pump inhibitors, which you saw above is a major contributor for SIBO. A review of research done in 2020 indicated that probiotics have a favorable effect on GERD.[87]

Standard treatment with PPIs not only causes more digestive problems, they also are simply not very effective. As a result, researchers continue to look for alternatives to this ailment that plagues up to 33% of Americans. A double-blind placebo-controlled human trial done in 2018 showed that patients who received two 500 mgs tablets of Amla berry twice per day had significantly improved GERD symptoms.[88]

If you go to the doctor to get help with your GERD, it is highly unlikely that he or she will prescribe stress management - even though stress is a major contributor to the illness.

A 2012 study concluded that "Reflux esophagitis is significantly associated with psychosocial stress, and the severity of reflux esophagitis correlates with the degree of stress." This is not new information. In 1993 the National Institutes of Health (NIH) published a paper stating that anxiety increases symptoms and severity for GERD patients, and that using anxiety reducing medication may help. I find it interesting that instead of suggesting more stress management techniques they recommend yet another medication that has already been shown to have a negative impact on gut microbiome.[89]

Perhaps we need to give more credit to the impact of stress on our gut health and do more to address it.[90]

Constipation is broadly defined as an unsatisfactory defecation characterized by infrequent stools, difficult stool passage or both. This often leads to the chronic use of laxatives. Laxatives have been shown to negatively impact the microbiome, which may make constipation worse yet users may become "addicted" to using laxatives as their own body unlearns how to normally expel fecal matter.[91]

A brand new study published in 2021 in *Frontiers in Cellular Infection and Microbiology* studies the microbiome of women with and without constipation. The overall composition of the gut microbiota changed in constipated women of reproductive age, characterized by a loss in *proteobacteria* and an increase in *bacteroidetes*. So if we go back to what we know about the microbiome, the solution is more about stress and food than taking laxatives.[92]

In an interesting article by Dr. Ray Peat, he discusses inflammation of the colon as a major contributor to chronic constipation. With an inflamed colon, many fiber sources often recommended will only make constipation worse. Instead, Dr. Peat recommends using Cascara Sagrada for its emodin content to reduce inflammation and allow contents to move freely through the bowels.[93]

Peptic ulcers are extremely common in the US as about 10% of the population has duodenal ulcers. *H Pylori* is the main cause of gastrointestinal ulcers.[94]

Eradicating *H Pylori* has been an effective way to treat ulcers. Some studies suggest that probiotics may be an effective strategy for resolving the dysbiosis that encourages *H Pylori* infection.[95]

Obviously digestive health has been very important for me since my bout with ulcerative colitis is what started me on this journey to learn about gut health. What always pains me is to see that most people's lives are deeply impacted by digestive disorders, yet doctors rarely give credence to that. They are very good at prescribing drugs in most cases, yet almost never teach people how to eat in a way that will alleviate these issues. This is one of my business goals moving forward, to partner with physicians that actually WANT to help their patients get better by making the necessary diet and lifestyle choices to heal. It certainly can be done and with little to no side effects or risk.

---

[76] https://gut.bmj.com/content/48/1/132
[77] https://www.ncbi.nlm.nih.gov/pmc/articles/PMC5757125/
[78] https://www.ncbi.nlm.nih.gov/pmc/articles/PMC6567822/
[79] https://www.frontiersin.org/articles/10.3389/fmed.2018.00304/full
[80] https://www.ncbi.nlm.nih.gov/pmc/articles/PMC5757125/
[81] https://www.niddk.nih.gov/health-information/digestive-diseases/crohns-disease/symptoms-causes
[82] https://www.sciencedaily.com/releases/2012/09/120913123512.htm
[83] https://www.ncbi.nlm.nih.gov/pmc/articles/PMC6039952/
[84] https://www.science.org/doi/10.1126/scitranslmed.aaf6397
[85] https://www.ncbi.nlm.nih.gov/pmc/articles/PMC2890937/
[86] https://www.ncbi.nlm.nih.gov/pmc/articles/PMC3099351/
[87] https://www.ncbi.nlm.nih.gov/pmc/articles/PMC7019778/
[88] https://pubmed.ncbi.nlm.nih.gov/29526236/
[89] https://pubmed.ncbi.nlm.nih.gov/8420248/
[90] https://www.ncbi.nlm.nih.gov/pmc/articles/PMC3576549/
[91] https://www.ncbi.nlm.nih.gov/pmc/articles/PMC4951383/
[92] https://www.frontiersin.org/articles/10.3389/fcimb.2020.557515/full
[93] http://raypeat.com/articles/articles/cascara-energy-cancer-fda-laxative-abuse.shtml
[94] https://www.medscape.com/answers/181753-13866/what-is-the-prevalence-of-peptic-ulcer-disease-pud-in-the-us
[95] https://www.ncbi.nlm.nih.gov/pmc/articles/PMC6151681/

SIX: HORMONES AND THE GUT

Hormones are a very complicated part of health. When they are balanced, we feel happy, energized, have good sleep and a strong libido. The hormones estrogen, progesterone, testosterone and cortisol are all closely interrelated and are strongly connected to gut health. Unfortunately, many people become estrogen dominant due to an overload of toxins that bind to estrogen receptors as well as the body's inability to detoxify it.

The gut contains microbes that produce an enzyme that metabolizes estrogens, called beta-glucuronidase. When these microbes are impaired, the enzyme is reduced and that process of eliminating estrogens is reduced allowing estrogen to build up in the body. As estrogen builds up this causes other estrogen-related problems, symptoms, and diseases.

A 2017 paper lists the following diseases as estrogen dependent outcomes: obesity, metabolic syndrome, cancer, endometrial hyperplasia, endometriosis, polycystic ovary syndrome, fertility, cardiovascular disease (CVD) and cognitive function.[96]

Another area of concern is estrogen dependent breast cancer. The estrogen-like compounds called xenoestrogens may promote the proliferation of certain species of bacteria that promote breast cancer.[97]

Progesterone opposes estrogen and we make less of it as we age, which increases our likelihood of becoming estrogen dominant. A study done in 2019 found that progesterone regulates the microbial composition of bacteria during pregnancy in a way that may help the baby develop. The researchers stated that *bifidobacterium* senses and responds to progesterone.[98]

A study done on rats found therapeutic benefit of post-TBI progesterone injections which might be due to its inhibitory effects on intestinal anti-inflammatory compounds related to cancer (NF-κB) and proinflammatory cytokines expression. This study is relevant to gut health because serious trauma and shock may initiate intestinal problems such as increased intestinal permeability (leaky gut) and translocation of intestinal bacteria and endotoxins.[99]

Testosterone is also affected by the gut microbiome. A 2019 study published in *Research in Biology* revealed that men and women with more gut bacteria diversity had higher levels of testosterone.[100]

Melatonin is considered the "sleep" hormone even though it has many other functions such as detoxification of free radicals, bone formation, and body mass regulation. The pineal gland is known as the source of the hormone, but the gut has 400 times more melatonin than the pineal gland! In fact, most melatonin receptors are found in the ileum and colon.

A 2011 study looked at the melatonin levels of patients with IBS, inflammatory bowel disease, and colorectal cancer. Supplements of melatonin improved pain for patients with lower bowel diseases. It also found that melatonin improved outcomes for cancer patients undergoing chemotherapy. The most interesting information I found in this research however, was that although many people are familiar with the idea that melatonin regulates circadian rhythms, it may not be the way you think.

Sleep cycles and melatonin are regulated to some extent through the pineal gland and light exposure, however it is predominantly regulated through the gut depending on what you eat and how well you digest it, rather than light. Don't throw out your blue blockers just yet though, you do still get some benefit by reducing blue light for regulating sleep, just not to your gut where most melatonin is made.[101]

Serotonin is another hormone very dependent on gut health in fact 90% of it is produced in the gut. Interestingly, drugs that target serotonin for depression have a major impact on the gut microbiome, bringing up the questions as to whether microbial interactions with antidepressants have consequences for health and disease.[102]

Some sources say that serotonin is actually the cause of depression rather than the cure and that it is made as a result of undigested materials in the gut-producing endotoxins. The intestines contain about 95% of the body's serotonin and having excess estrogens blocks the body's ability to break it down and excrete it.[103]

Insulin is the hormone that is made by the pancreas and is in charge of regulating the amount of glucose in the bloodstream by pushing glucose into the cells. A human study on urban Nigerians published in 2020 found Type 2 diabetes is associated with changes in the composition of the microbiome which suggests the connection with insulin regulation. More research needs to happen to learn how insulin and related diseases can be mitigated with gut health.[104]

Ghrelin & Leptin are your appetite and satiety hormones. Ghrelin signals to us we are hungry, leptin tells us when we have had enough to eat. A 2017 study done on humans with *H Pylori* found that when they treated them with amoxicillin they found that their ratio of *bacteroidetes* to *firmicutes* was changed to a higher proportion of *bacteroidetes:firmicutes* and also showed a decrease in ghrelin levels. This is interesting because higher *firmicutes* have been associated with lower rates of obesity.[105][106]

Having the right gut microbe balance can also affect your leptin levels that signal satiety. In a study done with mice researchers compared the microbiomes of conventional mice to sterilized mice and found the microbiome reduces the expression of neuropeptides that suppress body fat and that body fat inducing gut microbes are associated with leptin resistance.[107]

Cortisol is very well known for its presence when we are under stress and it is the body's main stress hormone. It helps us to utilize our macronutrients, reduce inflammation, influences sleep and wake cycles and can increase glucose to meet energy demands as needed as in the "fight or flight" response. A 2017 review on stress and the gut brain axis found that "Diet is one of the most important modifying factors of the microbiota-gut-brain axis." It goes on to say that alterations of the gut microbiome early in life due to antibiotics, lack of breastfeeding, stress and environmental factors can result in long term effects on stress-related physiology.[108]

It seems that cortisol is less affected by the gut, but that the gut is very much affected by cortisol. There are many studies demonstrating the damaging effects of stress on the body. In one that specifically covers the effect on the gut, researchers said they believe that gut inflammation leads to the activation of the HPA axis (discussed in Part 2, Chapter 3). They go on to say that the HPA axis is activated by microbiota-driven inflammation. Clearly inflammation is damaging our guts but may also be a driver of stress.[109]

Oxytocin is a neuropeptide made in the hypothalamus. It is often referred to as the "love" hormone. It is involved with bonding and is present during childbirth, breastfeeding and during sexual activity. In general, it is associated with feelings of physical and mental wellbeing. Although this hormone is not made in the gut, it does have some interesting connections to the microbiome. It has been shown to increase in the presence of lactobacillus reuteri from human breast milk. Researchers believe there is an opportunity to boost the gut microbes as a way to increase oxytocin levels to improve health issues such as immune dysfunctions, mental illness, metabolic diseases and even cancers.[110]

Vitamin D is actually not a vitamin D at all, but rather a prohormone according to researchers at the Hormone Health Network. It is produced by the kidneys to control the calcium levels in the blood. When the sun hits your skin, it produces cholecalciferol, which is then converted via the liver to calcidiol and then on to the kidneys which converts it yet again into the hormone used by the body called calcitriol.[111]

This hormone then binds to a protein that is present in every cell. Having low levels of vitamin D is associated with immune dysfunction, mental illness, infections and cardiovascular disease. Deficiencies in vitamin D are also associated with altered gut microbiome and mucosal layer of the intestinal.

According to a 2020 study published in *Frontiers in Immunology*, "If the mucus layer is breached, a single layer of intestinal epithelial cells acts as the next line of defense." As you can imagine, this leaves the body extremely vulnerable to pathogens and toxins that could pass through the tight junctions of the gut lining. There is a strong connection between alterations in gut microbiome of gut lining dysfunction with various autoimmune and immune system conditions. To sum things up, vitamin D is needed to maintain the gut lining, which once breached opens the doors to numerous illnesses.[112]

The thyroid hormones T4 and T3 regulate body temperature, metabolism, heart rate and are critical to overall health and especially to metabolic functions. The hormone triiodothyronine is referred to as T3 and thyroxine is referred to as T4. The thyroid releases T4 and it is converted in the liver and gut into T3, which is mainly what the body uses by absorbing from the bloodstream and sending it to the gut within the bile. The gut itself is a reservoir for thyroid hormones, especially T3. When the gut is inflamed the conversion of T4 to T3 is impaired and may result in hypothyroidism.[113]

Another study done in 2019 analyzing the stool samples of 74 patients with thyroid cancer, thyroid nodules and healthy control subjects indicated that dysbiosis of the gut microbiome was related to thyroid nodules and thyroid cancer whereas control subjects had healthy microbiomes.[114]

Hormones have been something I have worked a lot on for myself in the last few years. I turned 47 this year and have focused on the importance of balancing estrogen and testosterone for so many reasons. As we age the accumulation of estrogens can cause an array of problems and diseases. We need to make an effort to keep that in check. We also need to maintain a healthy thyroid to help us do that, along with many other functions of thyroid. Hormones can make the difference between being overweight or not, having a mental illness or not and even getting cancer or not. We can start with addressing diet and stress.

[96] https://pubmed.ncbi.nlm.nih.gov/28778332/

[97] https://pubmed.ncbi.nlm.nih.gov/30110974/

[98] https://www.sciencedaily.com/releases/2019/04/190416132129.htm

[99] https://www.ncbi.nlm.nih.gov/pmc/articles/PMC2222592/

[100] https://pubmed.ncbi.nlm.nih.gov/30940469/

[101] https://www.ncbi.nlm.nih.gov/pmc/articles/PMC3198018/

[102] https://www.sciencedaily.com/releases/2019/09/190906092809.htm

[103] http://raypeat.com/articles/articles/serotonin-disease-aging-inflammation.shtml

[104] https://www.frontiersin.org/articles/10.3389/fcimb.2020.00063/full

[105] https://www.ncbi.nlm.nih.gov/pmc/articles/PMC7285218/

[106] https://bmjopengastro.bmj.com/content/4/1/e000182

[107] https://academic.oup.com/endo/article/154/10/3643/2423894

[108] https://www.ncbi.nlm.nih.gov/pmc/articles/PMC5736941/

[109] https://www.ncbi.nlm.nih.gov/pmc/articles/PMC5794709/

[110] https://www.sciencedirect.com/science/article/pii/S2451965021000545

[111] www.hormone.org
[112] https://www.ncbi.nlm.nih.gov/pmc/articles/PMC6985452/
[113] https://www.ncbi.nlm.nih.gov/books/NBK500006/
[114] https://pubmed.ncbi.nlm.nih.gov/30584647/

SEVEN: SLEEP, IMMUNE SYSTEM & INFLAMMATION

According to the Centers for Disease Control and Prevention, approximately 70 million Americans have chronic sleep problems.[115]

One of the most underrated components of health and healing is sleep. Sleep is the time that our body repairs and heals itself. Several studies support the associations among sleep, immune function, and inflammation and patients with both inactive and active IBD have self-reported sleep disturbance. Sleep is considered to be an active state with restorative properties. Our sleep cycles, known as the circadian rhythm, are controlled by "clocks" within the brain and gut. When there are alterations in the brain such as stress, or in the gut such as GI problems, sleep problems can occur.[116]

A 2004 study found that IBS was significantly more common in those with sleep disturbances.[117]

In animal studies, researchers have found that when mice are subjected to alternating light and dark periods of circadian disruption they have a dramatic increase in the progression of the colitis.[118]

Sleep is critical to health, and not only will not getting enough sleep make it difficult to heal, it may also increase your risk of gut health problems.

Inflammation is the root of gut damage, as the lining first becomes inflamed before the tight junctions open up creating a leaky gut situation. There are many ways to control inflammation in the body. Stress reduction is a big one because of its effect on the vagus nerve (see Part 2, Chapter 10) and increased cortisol effects throughout the body. Inflammation can be reduced through diet, stress management, fasting and plant medicines. My favorite herb for reducing inflammation in the gut is berberine.

Inflammation is also caused by toxins that get into our body from food, water, air, or the skin. I recommend going through your skin care products and eliminating anything with synthetic chemicals. This seems drastic but is necessary to reduce the toxic burden to our bodies and hopefully reduce inflammation. Remove chemicals from your home such as cleaning agents, air fresheners and other products that contain chemicals. You will find there are literally hundreds of products with chemicals that you encounter every day.

Cells in the lining of the gut spend their lives excreting massive quantities of antibodies into the gut. The majority of your immune function is actually inside the gastrointestinal tract. When the lining of the gut or the gut microbiome is disrupted, immune system dysfunction can occur. The microbes within the gut are complicated and interact with various pathways and enzyme actions throughout the body that are still being studied. What is clearly understood is that the gut microbiome impacts multiple functions such as sleep patterns, nutritional response, metabolism and immunity. When sleep patterns are disrupted, the body becomes less resilient to stress and the stress hormone cortisol is increased.[119]

The intestinal tract is home to many microbes and is an active immunological organ, with more resident immune cells than anywhere else in the body. The gut microbiome is what allows us to endure infections and environmental stressors.[120]

The health of gut lining and microbiome balance are also related to cancer. When the lining or barrier of the gut is disturbed, inflammation and related diseases including cancer can occur. The lining of the gut is also responsible for detecting and eliminating invading bacteria.[121]

It is estimated that 20% of tumors are driven by microbes. Some tumors have been successfully treated with antibiotics demonstrating their bacterial origin.[122]

A 2009 study published in the *BMJ* showed that mice treated with prebiotic fiber had lower levels of lipopolysaccharides and inflammatory cytokines with less inflammation and oxidative stress. The reduced inflammation was associated with less gut permeability (leaky gut) and a stronger gut wall. Prebiotics are a fiber found in foods that feed beneficial bacteria.[123]

Chronic inflammation, a driver of many diseases, originates in the gut. When the gut lining is compromised creating dysfunction in the intestinal barrier, chronic low grade inflammation is induced in the gut and other organs. This barrier protects the other layers of the intestines and regulates the pro-inflammatory molecules and toxins from passing into the bloodstream.[124][125]

Low grade inflammation, regardless of location or severity, can impair digestion, absorption and gut motility as well as lead to gut lining permeability due to proinflammatory cytokines.[126]

Inflammation is clearly detrimental to the gut and overall health, but there are options. Both diet and supplements can help reduce inflammation. In human trials, probiotics showed benefit in reducing inflammation especially in subjects with bowel related inflammatory conditions.[127]

Let's not forget that stress is a major driver of inflammation as are the toxic food additives and processed foods that most people consume every single day. We can do better. Changing our daily habits only takes a little time and effort to make a difference.

---

[115] www.cdc.gov

[116] https://www.ncbi.nlm.nih.gov/pmc/articles/PMC3995194/

[117] https://pubmed.ncbi.nlm.nih.gov/15595333/

[118] https://pubmed.ncbi.nlm.nih.gov/18843092/

[119] https://www.nature.com/articles/s41422-020-0332-7

[120] https://www.ncbi.nlm.nih.gov/pmc/articles/PMC7587753/#bib58

[121] https://www.ncbi.nlm.nih.gov/pmc/articles/PMC7587753/#bib58

[122] https://onlinelibrary.wiley.com/doi/10.1002/path.5047

[123] https://gut.bmj.com/content/gutjnl/58/8/1091.full.pdf

[124] https://www.ncbi.nlm.nih.gov/pmc/articles/PMC5988153/

[125] https://www.ncbi.nlm.nih.gov/pmc/articles/PMC7231157/

[126] https://www.ncbi.nlm.nih.gov/pmc/articles/PMC2835780/

[127] https://www.ncbi.nlm.nih.gov/pmc/articles/PMC3257638/

EIGHT: NUTRIENT ABSORPTION, METABOLISM & WEIGHT LOSS

The small intestine is where most nutrient absorption happens. Your body absorbs the molecules from the food through the intestinal wall and into the bloodstream. If the small intestine is inflamed the process may be impaired and less nutrients will be absorbed.[128]

Less research has been done specifically on the absorption of nutrients, however a 2011 paper published in *Biochemistry Journal* shows that enzymes needed for absorption in the gut of water-soluble vitamins ascorbate, biotin, folate, niacin, pantothenic acid, pyridoxine, riboflavin, and thiamin are made by the microbiota of the gut, which if altered can diminish the enzymes needed for absorption.[129]

Gut health is linked to metabolic syndrome. Taking prebiotics, probiotics, and practicing dietary interventions has been effective in treating components or complications of metabolic syndrome such as energy balance, metabolic processes and by altering inflammatory signaling pathways and the immune system.[130]

Diet is one of the most important determinants of microbial diversity within the gut. A recent study comparing the gut microbiome of rural children in Burkina Faso with children in Italy showed that *bacteroidetes* were far more abundant in the microbiomes of African children and that the specific types that were increased were well suited to harvest energy from their plant-rich diet. Prebiotics are nondigestible substances that, when ingested, stimulate microbial growth of specific bacteria within the colon, particularly *bifidobacteria* and *lactobacilli*, that are associated with health benefits to the host. The prebiotics most commonly studied in the area of weight regulation are oligofructose and inulin.[131]

A 2018 study done on mice found that those who were obese had more gut dysbiosis than those of a normal weight. The researchers stated that obesity impacted cellular turnover, increased cell death which is associated with increased gut permeability.[132]

Weight loss has a lot to do with your gut bacteria balance and makeup. Short chain fatty acids (SCFA) are made in the gut with the help of dietary fibers. Adipocytes, or fat cells sense the increase of SCFA levels produced by intestinal microbe fermentation and respond by inducing leptin production. Leptin signals the brain to regulate appetite and energy expenditure, sending the signal to the brain that you have had enough to eat. If microbes are out of balance, the signal might not make it to the brain causing one to consistently overeat.[133]

Some studies have demonstrated a significant increase in the ratio of *firmicutes* to *bacteroidetes* in the obese microbiome of humans and mice.[134]

Microbes in intestines impact the absorption, breakdown, and storage of nutrients from the foods we consume. The type of food we eat is apparently just as important as the number of calories we consume when it comes to obesity and weight loss.[135]

A 2019 article in *Frontiers in Physiology* stated that cells within the gut responsible for making and secreting hormones have important roles in metabolism such as insulin sensitivity, glucose tolerance, fat storage, and appetite. Bacteria in the gut can also influence the hormones within the gut.[136]

A 2020 study on 14 men and 44 women taking part in a retail weight loss program which provided all meals concluded that contribution of the gastrointestinal microbiota as well as sex and body composition differences toward differential weight-reduction.[137]

Another paper that reviewed multiple studies showed that probiotics led to a significant decrease in BMI compared to placebo, however prebiotics had very little impact on BMI.[138]

Research done with monkeys fed with a Mediterranean diet that had lower body fat had higher amounts of *lactobacillus* animalis than higher body fat monkeys. In addition, monkeys fed a Western diet that were higher in body fat had more *ruminococcus champaneliensis* bacteria than lower body fat monkeys.[139]

Lactobacillus bacteria has been associated with lower body fat in previous studies.[140]

Another human study found that obese individuals were more likely to have a leaky gut (gut permeability) however that improved once they reached a healthy weight.[141]

Many of the clients who come to me ask for help with weight loss plus other issues like acne or joint pain. My approach is different, however. If we work on getting the best nutrition possible, eating the right foods at the right time, not only do we have the best shot of being as healthy as possible, we set ourselves up for success to find a healthy weight. It is very doable for each person, and there is really no reason for any person in America to be lacking in nutrition or being overweight. In fact, most of the diseases we suffer from are diseases of EXCESS due to overconsumption, yet these same people are deficient in many nutrients. Nutrition is king!

[128]https://www.ncbi.nlm.nih.gov/pmc/articles/PMC2835780/
[129]https://www.ncbi.nlm.nih.gov/pmc/articles/PMC4049159/
[130] https://pubmed.ncbi.nlm.nih.gov/26916014/
[131]https://www.ncbi.nlm.nih.gov/pmc/articles/PMC3601187/
[132]https://www.hindawi.com/journals/jdr/2018/3462092/#abstract
[133]https://www.ncbi.nlm.nih.gov/pmc/articles/PMC3601187/
[134]https://www.ncbi.nlm.nih.gov/pmc/articles/PMC3601187/
[135]https://www.ncbi.nlm.nih.gov/pmc/articles/PMC7333005/
[136]https://www.frontiersin.org/articles/10.3389/fphys.2019.00428/full
[137]https://www.ncbi.nlm.nih.gov/pmc/articles/PMC7463616/
[138]https://www.ncbi.nlm.nih.gov/pmc/articles/PMC5867888/
[139]https://microbiomejournal.biomedcentral.com/articles/10.1186/s40168-021-01069-y
[140]https://www.ncbi.nlm.nih.gov/pmc/articles/PMC4761174/
[141]https://academic.oup.com/ajcn/article/105/1/127/4637482

NINE: BONE, JOINT, LUNG AND ORAL HEALTH

At this point, you probably won't be surprised when I say there is also a cartilage-microbiome axis. It turns out that the gut microbiome in human cartilage suggests trafficking of bacteria between the gut and bone marrow. Researchers believe this is affected by regulation of nutritional absorption, regulation of the immune system at the gut endothelium, and translocation of microbes and molecular products of bacteria across the endothelial barrier and into the systemic circulation according to a 2018 study.[142]

Animal models have shown a relationship between microbiome makeup and bone and cartilage where the microbiome affects the amount of bone and bone quality. Preliminary studies show a relationship between the gut and osteoarthritis and osteoporosis.[143]

A healthy gut will absorb the right amount of calcium to keep bones healthy. Prebiotic fibers help to produce short chain fatty acids that increase calcium absorption and reduce risk for bone loss.[144]

It's hard for most people to think that changing their diet could alter their joint pain, but this in fact is the case. A human cohort study found that large amounts of the streptococcus species was associated with increased knee pain demonstrating that chronic knee pain could be addressed by improving the microbiome. This is important because many people treat their pain with NSAIDS, however those have also been shown to reduce beneficial bacteria in the microbiome which may further exacerbate joint pain.[145]

We have covered previously how antibiotics impact the gut microbiome and resulting disease. A study published in the *European Respiratory Journal* in 2018 was the first evidence to establish what is now referred to as the gut-lung axis. By using the gut-specific antibiotics on the lung confirm the presence of a functional gut-lung axis. It has been previously shown that those who receive antibiotics early in life have a much greater chance of developing asthma later in life.[146]

More research has been done on the effects of microbiome health on respiratory conditions. A 2020 review of research found that gut dysbiosis impacts the immunity of the lungs and subsequent respiratory diseases. Correlations were found between gut microbiome and asthma, chronic obstructive pulmonary disease, cystic fibrosis, lung cancer, and respiratory infections. Studies continue on the use of probiotics to treat these diseases via the gut.[147]

A 2020 study in *Cell: Trends In Cancer* describes the microbiome as "key modulators of both the carcinogenic process and the immune response against cancer."[148]

There is also an oral microbiome, which is closely connected to the lung microbiome. The oral microbiome is the second largest microbiome in the body second to the gut and includes seven hundred species of bacteria, fungi, as well as viruses (the same as other microbiomes in the body). The shift from healthy to disease-causing microorganisms within the oral microbiome leads to oral diseases like dental caries, periodontal disease, and cancer.[149][150]

Oral bacteria assist with colonizing the gut microbiome, however gut bacteria do not colonize the gut microbiome. Gum and periodontitis may affect the gut microbiome indicating treating the gut may help alleviate periodontal diseases.[151]

This year was an amazing year when it comes to research on gut health for lungs. As more research on COVID-19 unfolds, one paper which has gotten very little attention is of gut health and its effect on COVID-19 outcomes. I interviewed the author, Dr. Christine Bishara, and found she is a pioneer in the field of gut health as a way to prevent and treat our most common ailments. I hope other doctors will read her research and follow suit. I believe there are so many illnesses we can prevent if we take this simple but powerful approach.

[142] https://rmdopen.bmj.com/content/5/2/e001037
[143] https://www.ncbi.nlm.nih.gov/pmc/articles/PMC5737008/
[144] https://www.ncbi.nlm.nih.gov/pmc/articles/PMC4996260/
[145] https://www.nature.com/articles/s41467-019-12873-4
[146] https://erj.ersjournals.com/content/52/suppl_62/PA978
[147] https://www.ncbi.nlm.nih.gov/pmc/articles/PMC7415116/
[148] https://www.cell.com/trends/cancer/fulltext/S2405-8033(19)30265-1
[149] https://www.ncbi.nlm.nih.gov/pmc/articles/PMC6384374/
[150] https://www.ncbi.nlm.nih.gov/pmc/articles/PMC6503789/
[151] https://elifesciences.org/articles/45931

TEN: TAKING CONTROL OF YOUR HEALTH - STEPS TO HEALING

Many of the illnesses covered in this book are related to gut permeability or the leakiness of the gut. We know that that can happen as a result of stress, toxins, and the imbalance of gut microbiomes. With this knowledge, we can heal chronic diseases by first healing the gut lining and increasing beneficial bacteria.

The challenge comes for many people (like myself), who are so inflamed that eating foods high in fiber to feed bacteria come with digestive pain and irritation. In this case, we can first remove all fiber and other digestive irritants to allow the gut inflammation to calm down and heal. This approach worked very well for me and I use this with my clients with great success.

Step 1: Remove irritants that inflame the gut

It is strange for people to hear that they may need to omit legumes and leafy greens in order to heal their gut. These types of foods are seen as healthy for the gut, however for someone who is inflamed it might actually make things worse. Fiber is helpful to feed bacteria but it also needs to be digested.

If the gut lining is highly inflamed, sending fibrous foods through the intestinal tract can be compared to taking a brillo pad to a wound. It can irritate it even more. This may be why some people who eat legumes, grains, or vegetables experience digestive pain and bloating after eating.

The human gut should be able to deal with lectins, fibers, and other naturally occurring irritants, but the inflamed gut has low defenses and needs to be treated delicately. For this reason in the first stages of healing the gut, I recommend a fiber-free period. This means that one would exclude all fibers for a short period of time. Yes, that means removing all high fiber "healthy" foods including vegetables, leafy greens, grains, legumes, nuts, and seeds. This may seem extreme, but for serious inflammatory conditions it is often necessary.

Endotoxins are lipopolysaccharides that are bred within the gut as a gram-negative bacteria. The presence of endotoxins is added by overuse of antibiotics, increased incidence of Cesarean births, lack of breast-feeding, and reduced stomach acid due to use of proton-pump inhibitors.

Having LPS in the gut is quite normal but becomes problematic if the gut lining is permeable from having the tight junctions opening up and allowing endotoxins to pass the gut lining. PPIs are used to combat acid reflux conditions which can also be controlled with diet. By improving the stomach acids, we can improve digestion and reduce the growth of endotoxins.[152]

Chemicals that we get through food, water, air, and skin are also a concern. Food-borne chemicals called xenobiotics can also impair microbiome functions. Buying only organic foods, grass-fed meats, wild-caught fish and pasture raised eggs is a good start. We can also filter our water (I recommend the Berkey water filter system) and get fresh air every day.[153]

One of the worst chemicals in agriculture when it comes to gut health is glyphosate found in GMO and non-organic foods. Glyphosate is a pesticide that damages the gut linking by loosening its tight junctions causing leaky gut. Glyphosate also disrupts the microbiome and damages the gut lining even in small doses deemed safe by the FDA. *Roundup*, the brand name of glyphosate has also been implicated in many other diseases including celiac disease, ADHD, Alzheimer's disease, infertility and cancer. It is worth noting that glyphosate is often used on grains that are fed to animals, and animals are also susceptible to illness and disease from glyphosate. All animal products you consume should be organic, grass-fed animals not exposed to glyphosate.[154]

Even the quality of the air we breathe can affect our microbiome. Studies suggest a connection between particulate matter air pollution and gastrointestinal disease. In fact, air pollution has been linked to obesity and Type 2 diabetes due to its effects on the microbiome.[155]

Skin care products contain an alarming amount of gut disrupting chemicals. Cosmetics contain antimicrobials, parabens, phthalates, nanomaterials, and UV filters that can alter the microbiome.

Synthetic preservatives called parabens seem to worsen asthma in children and researchers believe that antimicrobial properties of parabens could promote an allergic reaction by altering the microbiome of the gut, respiratory tract, or both. Limiting exposure to synthetic ingredients in cosmetic and personal care products is a good way to reduce exposure to all chemicals.[156][157]

Removing all chemical toxins from personal care, foods, water and air by limiting exposure goes a long way to reduce the inflammation happening within the gut and the body. Medications are also common microbiome disruptors, so using natural remedies when possible is a good way to help protect the microbiome.

Step 2: Heal the gut lining

In order to heal the lining of the gut we must remove the things that are harming it (Step 1) and provide the body with necessary elements that support healing of tissue and reduction of inflammation.

Protein is always necessary for creating new tissue but there is a special kind of protein that has a magical healing effect on the gut. Gelatin is an animal protein from collagen that helps to rebuild hair, skin, nails and especially the gut lining. A recent publication shows that glycine alleviates colitis; but the use of gelatin, especially in the form of a concentrated gelatinous beef broth, for colitis, dysentery, ulcers, celiac disease, and other diseases of the digestive system, goes far back in medical history. http://raypeat.com/articles/articles/gelatin.shtml

Gelatin can be purchased as a supplement, or a cooking ingredient as in the popular kids snack, Jello. Gelatin is the cooked version of collagen, so using collagen from animals will provide the purest form of gelatin. Bones, skin, joints and feet all contain large amounts of collagen. All animals contain about 50% gelatin, and consuming animal organs such as the liver can also supply gelatin. I usually recommend people to make a large batch of soup with oxtail (beef tail) or chicken feet to drink a few days per week. Taking it before bed will also help you sleep and reduce any pain or discomfort you may have. Many people like to make or buy bone broth, but there may be some concerns with larger bones containing lead that would be present in the broth of the soup. Other ways to get gelatin would be making jello, ice cream and other concoctions or desserts. A short cut healing broth can be made by dissolving gelatin powder in water as the base for your soups and stews.

Glycine is an amino acid in gelatin. In a 2017 review, glycine cured epithelial damage by certain drugs used in research to cause inflammation. According to the report, glycine is protective against many intestinal disorders including gastric ulcers due to its cytoprotective and anti-inflammatory effect.[158]

Another very helpful amino acid is glutamine, the most abundant amino acid in the body used by intestinal cells. Glutamine promotes the growth of new gut lining cells, regulates the tight junctions of the gut and suppresses inflammation as well as protects cells against cellular stress. This was something I used regularly in my healing journey with colitis. It has no side effects, and can be safely taken in very large doses. Glutamine is found in cabbage and I have heard some people use the juice in their healing protocols but I simply took the powdered supplement and found it helpful.[159]

Step 3: Increase diversity of microbes

There is no specific microbiota composition that everyone needs to strive for other than having diversity of species and an appropriate balance of firmicutes, and bacteroidetes which make up about 90% of the microbiome. Each person will have a different set of microbes and still be healthy.

Dietary choices have a major impact on microbiome composition which influences numerous biological processes and the ability of the gut to make short chain fatty acids. When the microbiome is altered it can increase the risk of changes or damage to the mucus layer of the intestinal lining, leading to increased permeability and particles making their way through the lumen to the bloodstream.[160]

Short chain fatty acids are a subset of fatty acids created by the gut from fermentation of polysaccharides. SCFA are involved with regulation of metabolism, inflammation, and diseases and have anti-inflammatory, antitumorigenic, and antimicrobial effects; and alter gut integrity. Short chain fatty acids have been shown to have a beneficial effect on the gut-brain axis and play a role in mental health and brain functions. Needless to say, these fatty acids are critical to a healthy functioning gut.[161][162]

All foods affect the microbiota, however carbohydrates, proteins, and fats do have differing effects. Carbohydrates include both digestible and indigestible substrates. These carbohydrates contain digestible and indigestible fibers. Fermentable fibers are easily fermented by bacteria in the colon, while non-fermentable fibers are not. Fermentable fibers create SCFA such as butyrate which help to reduce risk for cancers, control appetite and increase transit time of foods. Prebiotic fibers are resistant to digestion and assist gut microbiota to metabolize into SCFAs.

Proteins affect the gut microbiome differently depending on the source of protein. For example, meat and dairy products have been shown to increase anaerobic bacteria which play a role in inflammatory conditions. Saturated fats were shown to be more conducive to dysbiosis than however a high omega-6/omega-3 polyunsaturated fats ratio has been related to an enhanced gut barrier permeability and metabolic endotoxemia.[163]

Plant fibers from both fruits and vegetables support the growth of beneficial bacteria if the gut can tolerate them. If not, you will need to start with less fibers until your gut is healthy enough to tolerate more. Polyunsaturated fats from omega 6 sources such as seed oils like canola oil should be limited in favor of omega 3 fatty fats such as fish oil. However, a 2020 study stated that it's not the fat that affects microbiome negatively on higher fat diets, it is the displacement of fiber. Lack of fiber is more the cause of dysbiosis than any detrimental effect from dietary fat.[164]

In working with many people with diverse microbiome issues, it has been my experience that people often have so much inflammation in the gut that they cannot tolerate many plant fibers. This can make it difficult to work on diversity of microbiome when nearly everything you eat causes bloating, gas and pain. For this reason, I recommend a low fiber diet for those with serious gut inflammation or disease. In fact, the worse the inflammation the less fiber that is tolerated.

After a period of a few weeks to a few months, depending on the person, plant fibers can then be reinstated back into the diet a little bit at a time. Fruits seem to be tolerated the best, so I often start there, then on to cooked vegetables, and lastly, but very conservatively, raw vegetables. I never recommend people add legumes or grains back into the diet because they almost always cause inflammation if consumed regularly.

Probiotics

Probiotics are defined as "living microorganisms, which when administered in adequate amounts confer health benefits on the host." Probiotics may induce changes in the intestinal microbiota and stabilize microbial communities. I personally had some good results using probiotics however by themselves it never lasted and ultimately would flare at some point until I went through the carnivore diet. The product I used is now called visbiome and can be found at www.visbiome.com and this product did show a higher rate of remission for ulcerative colitis patients as compared to patients that did not use it.[165][166]

A 2013 review stated that probiotics not only enhance barrier function by inducing synthesis and assembly of tight junctions, but also preventing disruption of tight junctions. Bioactive factors released by probiotics trigger activation of various cell signaling pathways that lead to strengthening of tight junctions and the barrier function.[167]

A 2003 article in the *BMJ* suggests that probiotics have a local and systemic anti-inflammatory effect by modulating flora by reducing proinflammatory cytokines.[168]

A 2004 double-blind placebo controlled crossover study done with children with dermatitis found that those given probiotics had improved gut health and resulted in better outcomes of dermatitis.[169]

Although not a probiotic, berberine is a bitter alkaloid from the barberry plant, oregon grape root or goldenseal plant that has been used in herbal medicine to improve gut health. A 2018 study on mice showed that berberine reduced intestinal tumors and restored gut microbiota. I take berberine every day as part of my gut health protocol.[170]

Berberine has been shown to be effective for use with hyperlipidemia, cancer, metabolic syndrome, polycystic ovarian syndrome, and liver disease by reducing pathogenic bacteria and increasing beneficial bacteria in the gut.[171] It also has beneficial effects on the immune cells of the intestinal immune system and affects the expression of several intestinal immune factors and is effective at reducing low-grade inflammation.[172]

Another study on berberine done one mice showed an increase in the microbe species *akkermansia* that improved atherosclerosis. *Akkermansia* is found in larger amounts in thinner people and is considered to be helpful for maintaining a healthy body weight.[173]

Food Choices

This is the biggest question I get from people who have inflammatory bowel disease or any kind of digestion problems. Most people are either eating a lot of processed foods or a lot of vegetables and high fiber foods. Unfortunately, food with a high residue that is difficult to digest can cause a lot of digestion problems. This often gets confused with what is healthy eating, because the public has been told for many years now that more vegetables equate to better health. Plant-based diets are also considered "healthy" because they omit saturated fats and replace them with polyunsaturated fats and seed oils that can cause a lot of inflammation.

Since we have discussed the importance of a diverse and balanced microbiome, we need to know how to feed it. Research points to higher fiber foods to help feed good bacteria in the gut. However, for people with inflammatory conditions or poor digestion, high fiber foods can be more problematic. All foods can feed bacteria, but eating foods that are easier to digest while nourishing the body and microbiome can be challenging.

According to Dr. Ray Peat, "The toxins of plants include phenols, tannins, lectins/agglutinins, and trypsin-inhibitors, besides innumerable more specific metabolic inhibitors, including "anti-vitamins." Unsaturated fats themselves are important defenses, since they inhibit trypsin and other proteolytic enzymes, preventing the assimilation of the proteins that are present in seeds and leaves, and disrupting all biological processes that depend on protein breakdown, such as the formation of thyroid hormone and the removal of blood clots." Therefore, vegetables, legumes, grains, nuts and seeds are all very problematic foods for the gut.[174]

Protein is fairly easy to digest for most people. You will need about .8 grams per kilogram of body weight or more to sustain the tissues of the body. For most people that means a minimum of 100grams. The best sources of protein that are easy to digest are animal proteins. Grass fed beef, wild caught fish and seafood, pasture raised poultry and eggs are good choices. If dairy bothers you, you may need more time healing the gut before including milk, however milk and cheese are good sources of protein and calcium. Plant based proteins such as soy, legumes, nuts, and seeds are very difficult to digest and high in lectins that can irritate and inflame the gut.

Carbohydrates are needed for fueling your body and for many metabolic processes. Even though I was successful at healing my gut using the carnivore diet, I do believe I would have done better had I included carbohydrates in an easy to digest form such as honey or juice. The body can make glucose from your protein, but it does this in the liver through a process called gluconeogenesis and it results in high stress hormone cortisol. This can negatively impact thyroid functions and cause increased inflammation in the body. By giving your body easy to digest carbohydrates, you provide the liver with the glucose necessary to convert thyroid hormones T4 into T3, the form most used in your body. Fruits and root vegetables such as potatoes and yams are the easiest to digest carbohydrates as opposed to grains or starches. Honey and fruit juice are good choices for people who have extremely sensitive stomachs such as Crohn's or ulcerative colitis patients.

Fats have been demonized for so long, most people are afraid to eat them. Even more so are the saturated fats. Some clinic studies indicate they are inflammatory, however it is the polyunsaturated fats that are less stable especially when exposed to heat. Saturated fats from animal proteins or coconut oil are the safest for the gut and the entire body. Seed oils such as canola oil are highly toxic and should be avoided.

When I was in graduate school in 2001 we studied epidemiology and public health. One study on fats and health that no student will forget is the Framingham Heart Study. This is a cohort study done over the course of many years, to demonstrate the dangers of saturated fats and other health information. It turns out that the long-running study was never able to connect saturated fats to heart disease, so the study was buried for many years as it was a research flop. Research continues to debunk the fears that saturated fats cause heart disease and cancer.[175]

Another study, the *Minnesota Coronary Study* conducted human research between lower fat and higher fat diets finding no difference in outcomes for cardiovascular disease, cardiovascular deaths and total mortality.[176]

Finally, a 2018 review stated that no evidence exists that saturated fats cause harm and that they are actually helpful for Type 2 Diabetes and the article points out that it is the processed foods that do more harm in terms of cardiovascular disease.[177]

There is no reason to avoid animal foods from a health standpoint. Saturated fats are healthy for the body and are naturally occurring in most animal proteins so there is no need to add additional fats. All of the nutrients needed by the body can be found in meat, dairy, eggs, fish and seafood. With the addition of fruits, you will get all the nutrients you need.

It was my experience that eating a low fiber and low residue diet to include animal proteins and broths with gelatin was the most helpful in reducing irritation and symptoms. This can be followed up with juice or honey, and fruits that are easy to digest such as melon until the person can tolerate more foods without symptoms. Adding foods back into the diet should be a slow and gradual process.

Stress

As you have read in Part 1, stress is a major inducer of autoimmune disease. For me it was a death, divorce, move, and job change that ultimately put me in a state of chronic stress. Each person has a different set of stressors and in Part 1 I explained how stress affects the body and specifically the gut. We know that the gut and mind are connected through the gut-brain axis, so if we want to take care of the gut, we cannot ignore the importance of emotional well being.

Evaluating the stress in your life may be more challenging than you realize. We get very used to stress, especially if we live with it everyday. Being overworked, underrested, having worries about finances or relationships is very "normal" but the body is not designed to be in a constant stressed state.

Some things that were helpful for me in managing stress were counseling, having more fun, saying "no" more, getting more sleep and strengthening my friend/support network. I spent more time doing things I love like surfing or swimming, taking a lot of walks outdoors and going to bed early. Take every opportunity to have fun, laugh and be happy. These things increase oxytocin as the hormone antidote to cortisol, and we don't get enough of it.

Some people find benefits in meditation, however even as a yoga teacher, that was not something I did consistently. However, moving meditations like yoga, stretching and relaxing were a great stress relief. Whatever works to reduce your feelings of stress is fine, you don't need to adhere to some practice that doesn't resonate with you.

Stress can be from other sources besides emotional or mental challenges. Environmental toxins, not eating enough, too low of glucose, overexercising and electromagnetic fields (EMF) are all sources of stress that the body responds to with an increase in cortisol and inflammation. Humans are exposed to more stress now than ever before, and unfortunately it is considered very "normal."

The Vagus Nerve

Stress and trauma can have profound effects on the digestive system. When we are under stress our body has a physical response to it. We may feel mentally or emotionally stressed and have an increase in our stress hormones, our digestive fluids decrease, blood flow to extremities decrease, and blood sugar rises. The body does not know the difference between a lion chasing you and a bad driver cutting you off in traffic. It only knows your response. As Hans Selye said, "It's not the stress that kills us, it's the reaction to it."

When we have an emotional reaction to a stressor it activates the body to deal with a threat. These physiological changes are normal, but are only intended to last for a short period of time. For most people however, stress is now daily and sometimes throughout the day. It can be from worries about finances, too many responsibilities, relationship struggles or anything that upsets or worries you. Past traumas that are in our minds can have the same effect and more. Whatever puts the stressful thoughts in our minds will trigger the reaction in our body. The reaction runs from the nerves in the brain throughout the body, activating it to respond to the stressor (threat). That reaction is called the sympathetic nervous system. It puts our bodies in the best physical condition to withstand a fight or to flee, which is why it's called "fight or flight".

In a normal situation, that threat would pass, the body would return to the non-stressed state called parasympathetic state. This is where the body should remain MOST of the time. In the parasympathetic state the digestive processes are normal, blood flows to all of the organs as it should and the nerves from the brain send appropriate messages to all of the organs in the body. The parasympathetic state is alternatively referred to as the "rest, digest, and repair" state, since that is what occurs when you are in it.

The vagus nerve runs through the body and all of the digestive organs as well as immune organs like the thymus. As mentioned in Part 1, chronic stress or traumas - especially early life trauma - can damage the vagus nerve and affect the digestive processes, especially gut motility or the movement of food and stool through the digestive tract. Neurons are sent from a thought in the brain or some stimuli which send a signal through the length of the nerve, releasing neurotransmitters to necessary organs. Research has shown that the vagus nerve can reduce inflammation and alter your brain function and mood.[178]

Chronic stress or traumas can impair this messaging system. When we are under stress we breathe shallowly, using just our lungs and not engaging the diaphragm (belly) which unfortunately becomes a habit. Similar to a muscle in your body, the vagus nerve can lose its function (tone) and it's ability to signal the organs is reduced. It turns out that the function of the vagus nerve relies on your breathing so much that being stressed every day can result in malfunctioning organs and systems simply because of the mishap in messaging. In short, stress may be causing a problem with your organs in part because of nerve signaling issues.

A malfunctioning vagus nerve can result in gut irritation, constipation, diarrhea, food sensitivities, autoimmune disease, poor immune function, mental health disorders and general inflammation. This nerve plays a leading role in hearing, breathing, vocalizing, swallowing and other bodily functions that you never even think about. It also signals your heart, kidneys, liver, and gallbladder. The longest nerve in the body, it helps to control your hunger, blood sugar, and digestive fluids and functions because it runs through all of the organs related to digestion.

When the nerve cannot adequately signal its related organs, any of these problems can happen. So while choosing the right foods and eliminating toxins from your environment are important, it will not overcome dysfunctions caused by chronic stress or trauma. Traumas must be dealt with so that the body does not hold on to the stress of it and relearning how to breathe adequately in the face of stress is a big step in the right direction in fixing this portion of digestive malfunctions. This, I believe, is why yoga is so effective at reducing the effects of stress on the body. Yoga teaches a person how to breathe properly, and counteracts the effects of daily stress. Addressing traumas so that they are not recurring in your mind is an important step in healing the physical body from the constant reminder and reliving the trauma.

The vagus nerve is not part of diagnosis or treatment of any disease or condition within the Western medical model. Why? Because most doctors are not given any training on it in medical school and most don't understand the connection between stress or trauma and physical health problems, yet this is one of the main connection points.

Books I highly recommend are *The Body Keeps Score* for trauma survivors and *Activate Your Vagus Nerve* for an easy user guide on caring for this very important nerve. Also, to understand more about how stress affects you and how to control it, I recommend *Why Zebras Don't Get Ulcers*.

Managing stress is more than just keeping a positive attitude. It is the ACTIVE practice of proper breathing, controlling stressful thoughts, using your vagus nerve, connecting with others and ultimately reducing the amount of work and responsibilities in your life if they are causing you stress. You can create your own stress management practice like I do with my clients that include action items or a routine similar to your workout routine. This might include things like a breathing exercise, singing or humming, calling a friend or meeting with them in person, doing something creative that brings you happiness or even a cold shower! The point is, it will not happen if you are stuck in a pattern of overwork and overstress and do not take the time to care for yourself.

Fasting For Gut Health

Fasting seems to be a controversial topic. Some believe it is the Holy Grail to health, others believe it is too damaging. In my experience, it was very helpful so long as I did not fast too long too often. Fasting is the restriction of food or calories for a set period of time. There are many versions of fasting, including intermittent fasting, extended fasting, alternate day fasting and others.

The fasting that worked best for me and that I see people have the most success with is intermittent fasting. I did a few longer fasts for 24, 48 and 72 hours but I felt very stressed after the longer fasts and I do believe it can be harmful to the thyroid by increasing cortisol if practiced too often.

The most studied and easy to accomplish form of fasting is intermittent fasting in which one would reduce the time frame in which they eat. For example, if you had dinner at 7pm and woke up in the morning at 7am having had nothing in between, that would be a 12 hour fast. During this time your glucose will have been mostly depleted and the body will create ketones or use fat and protein for energy. The downside of this is that in the process of creating energy from protein and fat, stress hormones are created. Fasting too long or too often can create too high of cortisol and high cortisol effects such as impaired sleep or anxiety. Some people can fast in the morning or in the evening by having an earlier dinner and fasting until morning. Some people can fast in the morning and have dinner as normal, so as to improve sleep. There are many ways to fast but one should not ignore any ill effects such as anxiety or insomnia if you are fasting. Listen to your body, fasting is not for everyone.

Intermittent fasting has been shown to have a significant reduction in age-related pathologies and improved gut barrier function in studies done on fruit flies. Now, you are not a fruit fly, but this may suggest what could be possible for humans. In my experience, I saw great benefits to my gut health while practicing intermittent fasting as part of my overall protocol. Many other things need to be addressed, and fasting alone may not produce the result you are looking for but can be an excellent adjunct to a more comprehensive strategy.[179]

A study published in the *New England Journal of Medicine* in 2019 showed that a time-restricted eating window of six hours produced improved resiliency and reduced cancer and obesity risks. The authors state "most if not all organ systems respond to intermittent fasting in ways that enable the organism to tolerate or overcome the challenge and then restore homeostasis. Repeated exposure to fasting periods results in lasting adaptive responses that confer resistance to subsequent challenges." This means that your periods of fasting have benefits long after the fasting period ends. Also, the report suggests that fasting can improve body composition, reduce diabetes, improve cognitive functions, reduce the risk for cardiovascular disease and other obesity related illnesses.[180]

In other animal models, intermittent fasting was shown to improve the microbiome, reduce inflammation having a positive effect for multiple sclerosis.[181]

In a 2017 study, mice who had chemically induced colitis and fasted had an increase in epithelial cells and a decrease in inflammation.[182]

When you fast, the body makes beta hydroxybutyrate that helps to reduce inflammation. Fasting has also been shown to improve the microbiome. A small human study was done to investigate a seven day water only fast compared to a seven day juice fast. Water-only fasting dramatically changed the participants' gut bacteria and developed more homogenous gut microbiomes during the fasting period.[183]

Many people feel that healing their disease is impossible or that they are required to take medications to maintain their health. I believe this is false. I've experienced true healing using these methods myself. I've also witnessed it in others. I've seen people use gut health strategies to lose weight, balance hormones, heal thyroid diseases, cure acne, resolve mental illness, and solve tough digestive diseases. It really is possible, despite what you may have been told. Practice these methods and be patient, improvement in your gut health will come, and likely many other resolutions as well.

[152] https://www.ncbi.nlm.nih.gov/pmc/articles/PMC4566437/
[153] https://www.nature.com/articles/s41598-018-29376-9
[154] https://detoxproject.org/glyphosate/glyphosate-and-roundup-negatively-affect-gut-bacteria/
[155] https://pubmed.ncbi.nlm.nih.gov/29783199/
[156] https://www.ncbi.nlm.nih.gov/pmc/articles/PMC6691726/
[157] https://www.niehs.nih.gov/health/topics/agents/cosmetics/index.cfm
[158] https://www.ncbi.nlm.nih.gov/pmc/articles/PMC5350494/
[159] https://www.ncbi.nlm.nih.gov/pmc/articles/PMC5454963/
[160] https://www.ncbi.nlm.nih.gov/pmc/articles/PMC6835969/
[161] https://pubmed.ncbi.nlm.nih.gov/24388214/
[162] https://www.frontiersin.org/articles/10.3389/fendo.2020.00025/full
[163] https://www.ncbi.nlm.nih.gov/pmc/articles/PMC6835969/
[164] https://microbiomejournal.biomedcentral.com/articles/10.1186/s40168-020-0791-6
[165] https://journals.lww.com/md-journal/Fulltext/2018/12210/The_clinical_effects_of_probiotics_for.116.aspx
[166] https://www.ncbi.nlm.nih.gov/pmc/articles/PMC3539293/
[167] https://www.ncbi.nlm.nih.gov/pmc/articles/PMC3864899/
[168] https://gut.bmj.com/content/53/5/620
[169] https://pubmed.ncbi.nlm.nih.gov/15520759/
[170] https://pubmed.ncbi.nlm.nih.gov/30205580
[171] https://www.frontiersin.org/articles/10.3389/fcimb.2020.588517/full
[172] https://www.ncbi.nlm.nih.gov/pmc/articles/PMC7933196/
[173] https://pubmed.ncbi.nlm.nih.gov/29202334/
[174] http://raypeat.com/articles/articles/vegetables.shtml
[175] https://www.ncbi.nlm.nih.gov/pmc/articles/PMC4159698/
[176] https://pubmed.ncbi.nlm.nih.gov/2643423/
[177] https://pubmed.ncbi.nlm.nih.gov/30084105/
[178] https://pubmed.ncbi.nlm.nih.gov/24997031/
[179] https://www.ncbi.nlm.nih.gov/pmc/articles/PMC5988561/
[180] https://www.nejm.org/doi/full/10.1056/nejmra1905136

[181]https://www.ncbi.nlm.nih.gov/pmc/articles/PMC6460288/
[182]https://www.ncbi.nlm.nih.gov/pmc/articles/PMC5612824/
[183]https://www.sciencedirect.com/science/article/pii/S25900978
19300035

ELEVEN: PREPARE FOR SUCCESS

In order to be successful with changing your daily habits and setting yourself up for success you will need to plan ahead. This means planning your meals, stocking your refrigerator and pantry with helpful foods, getting rid of things that may cause inflammation to your body, and allowing yourself time for daily exercise and practicing daily resiliency exercises.

The lists below will help you create your plan and give you a starting point. Many of these things may be hard to implement if they are not your daily habit. The way to create new habits is to PRACTICE DAILY. Create your plan, follow it daily and soon it will all be second nature for you.

Foods

Animal Proteins

Grass fed land animals - beef, lamb, bison, pork, poultry

Wild caught fish and seafood - mahi, flounder, cod, halibut, salmon, scallops, clams, oysters, crab and lobster

Dairy - milk, cream, kefir, cottage cheese (without thickeners), cheese, goat or sheep milk and goat cheese, eggs

Fruits (juice only for people with active ulcerative colitis or Crohn's)

Organic berries, melon, papaya, pulp free juices, ripe banana, guava, passion fruits, fruits, pineapple and mangos.

If you have decent digestion you can add in peaches, pears, apples, and oranges

Vegetables (not for people with active ulcerative colitis or Crohn's)

Organic cucumbers (peeled), carrots, celery, radish, potatoes, sweet potatoes, green beans, asparagus, cooked squashes, and cooked mushrooms

Those with better digestion can have well cooked broccoli, cauliflower, and brussels sprouts

Grains, Legumes, Nuts and Seeds

All grains contain lectins and oxalates and are hard on digestion so I do not recommend eating them. This includes all wheat, rice, oats, barley, quinoa, kidney beans, garbanzo beans, navy beans, pinto beans, and lentils.

Nuts and seeds such as almonds, cashews, brazil nuts, sunflower seeds, chia seeds, and walnuts also contain lectins and oxalates and are best avoided.

Drinks

Fresh juices including pulp free orange juice, apple juice, and pomegranate juice are all safe for the gut so long as they do not contain particles.

Limit juice consumption if you have trouble regulating blood sugar and always consume fruit with protein.

Coffee is ok unless it gives you a negative effect. Sparkling waters are fine unless you have an autoimmune flare, in which case it may cause further bloating.

Alcohol can be very toxic to the gut (and all tissues) so I highly recommend avoiding it.

Helpful Gut Health Supplements (details of each are in Part 2, Chapter 10)

Berberine

Glutamine

Gelatin

Probiotics

Magnesium

Personal Care Products Detox

Remove all products with synthetic ingredients such as parabens, fragrances and preservatives. Assess all of your skin care, toiletries and home cleaning products. For more information on toxic skin care visit Environmental Working Group at www.ewg.org and search the databases for the products you are looking for.

Common toxic and hazardous ingredients

Includes preservatives, fragrances, and heavy metals. You may see them on labels listed as butylated hydroxyanisole (BHA) and butylated hydroxytoluene (BHT), formaldehyde & formaldehyde releasing agent, N-Ethylpentedrone (NEP) and N-Methyl-2-pyrrolidone (NMP), Oxybenzone, Parabens, Per- and poly-fluoroalkyl substances (PFAS), Phthalates, Siloxanes, Talc and Toluene.

Common beauty products that contain hazardous chemicals include:[184]

Aftershave balms

Bath soaps and shower gel

Body care products

Cosmetics

Creams and lotions

Deodorant

Eye drops

Hair conditioners

Hand soaps

Hygiene wash

Liquid formulations

Multi-purpose cleaners

Products for babies

Sunscreen

Toiletries

Create Your Stress Management Routine

Consider including meditations, breathing exercises and vagus nerve exercises into your daily routine. Shoot for at least one resiliency exercise per day. See the list below for ideas:

Meditation

Yoga

Walking meditation

Breathing exercises/diaphragmatic breathing

Singing/Humming/Gargling

Auricular acupuncture (or earlobe acupressure)

Massage and bodywork

Cognitive Behavioral Therapy

Hypnotherapy for PTSD

EFT Tapping

Create Your Exercise Routine

When the body is healing from a major inflammatory disease such as colitis, you may feel too tired to exercise. Movement still needs to happen, but it can be very gentle and relaxing. For people in this stage, I recommend daily walking, easy stretching, gentle yoga or pilates.

As you heal and gain strength and energy you can add more exercise. Overexercising can be very stressful on the body. Most of the overexercising I have seen that causes people trouble is excessive cardio. Light strength training produces more results with less stress. As you are able, you can incorporate 2-3 strength training days per week.

Create Your Sleep Routine

Sleep is a critical component of healing. Your body is in a parasympathetic state when we rest, digest, and repair. Most of us need 7-9 hours of uninterrupted sleep to feel rested and give our body the healing time it needs. If you have trouble falling or staying asleep, consider a bedtime routine that helps you reduce light exposure or having to use the restroom at night. Turn off electronic devices at least 2 hours before bed.

Remove stressful stimuli such as news or even books that evoke stressful thoughts. Dim the lights an hour or two before bed or use candles. Stop drinking liquids at least 1 hour before bed. Use a fan or other source of white noise to block out external sounds that can wake you up.

Supplements I have found helpful for sleep:

Magnesium

High calcium foods

CBD with CBN

Valerian root

Melatonin

I hope that sharing this research with you has given you faith and confidence in approaching your mystery illness through gut health. So much research is surfacing every year validating what the father of medicine, Hippocrates, taught so long ago. "All disease begins in the gut" and if we follow that rule of treating the gut as the cornerstone of our health, not only do we have a good chance at resolving health issues but we may just optimize our health and prevent illnesses in the future. This is true health and wellness, the prevention of illness by starting within ourselves

---

[184]https://www.researchgate.net/publication/271387744_Hazard ous_Ingredients_in_Cosmetics_and_Personal_Care_Products_an d_Health_Concern_A_Review

ACKNOWLEDGMENTS

Thank you to my family for their support through the years of struggle and study.

ABOUT THE AUTHOR

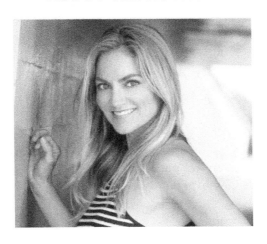

Nicole Carter is a Certified Health Education Specialist (CHES), corporate wellness consultant, and health coach with over 18 years of experience in health and wellness who is passionate about empowering people to take control of their health. Because of her holistic expertise, Nicole has been a guest speaker at International Conferences, Medical Conferences, University Conventions, local and national news networks, radio programs, and Internet shows. Nicole has been featured on International News Channels such as the BBC.

Please leave your honest review on Amazon.com / Goodreads / your local Amazon site

To learn more about how to work with Nicole please visit

healthywithnicole.com

Find Nicole @

Goodreads Nicole_Carter

Facebook healthywithnicolecarter

Instagram /healthy_with_nicole

Twitter NicoleCarter100

YouTube HealthyWithNicole

For physicians or groups interested in offering holistic health education to patients or employees please visit www.thewellnessexperienceonline.com

Made in the USA
Columbia, SC
28 November 2023

27226700R00098